Every week Elle Halliwell keeps millions of Australians up to date on all things entertaining and stylish thanks to her work with the country's top media outlets.

With more than a decade's experience in print and television media, the Australian journalist has become one of the country's favourite showbiz and fashion commentators, reporting beauty, style and celebrity news via her weekly columns in *The Daily* and *Sunday Telegraph*s and number one national radio show, Confidential on Nova.

Elle Halliwell
A MOTHER'S CHOICE

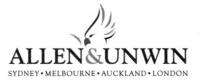

ALLEN&UNWIN
SYDNEY·MELBOURNE·AUCKLAND·LONDON

First published in 2018

Allen & Unwin
83 Alexander Street
Crows Nest NSW 2065
Australia
Phone: (61 2) 8425 0100
Email: info@allenandunwin.com
Web: www.allenandunwin.com

A catalogue record for this book is available from the National Library of Australia

ISBN 978 1 76063 277 9

Set in 13.5/17 pt Granjon by Midland Typesetters
Printed and bound in Australia by Griffin Press

10 9 8 7 6 5 4 3 2 1

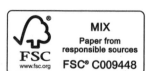

The paper in this book is FSC® certified. FSC® promotes environmentally responsible, socially beneficial and economically viable management of the world's forests.

To my boys

Contents

Happy New Year!

1 January 2016

On New Year's Day I was head-butted by a giant toucan. Its hot, vinyl beak made a sucking sound as it stuck to my bare back, which had started turning pink in the hot sun. I peeled myself free and swam to the other side of the pool—which was only a single breaststroke away from my original spot. The giant inflatable bird had been a ridiculous idea, considering our temporary pool could barely fit more than four comfortably *without* blow-up wildlife.

My husband Nick had disregarded the instructions to set up the plastic dipping pool on a flat surface, and now it threatened to dump its 2000-litre contents onto the lawn as my girlfriends and I lazed around its plastic periphery. It was a novel way to ease our New Year's Eve hangovers and keep us from cooking beneath the mid-summer sun. Nick was the only one of our little group who seemed unscathed by the previous night's frivolities.

Our good friends Mike and Briana, and my sister-in-law Chrissy and her husband Angus, had spent the night with us at Nick's parents' house. We had just moved into a self-contained apartment below their home in Sydney's inner west in a bid to save up a bigger deposit for our first home. Their place was the perfect party house. Nick's mum Het, in a stroke of genius, had two dishwashers installed in the kitchen to cater for parties when they built the house, and it boasted a huge balcony with views over Sydney Harbour's Cockatoo Island—one of the launch spots for the New Year's Eve fireworks.

The plan was to pop a few bottles of champagne and retire just after midnight to make sure we were all fresh and fired up for lunch the next day. It had become a tradition amongst our close friends that we would celebrate the *beginning* of the New Year, rather than the end of the previous one. There were exceptions, but most of us would rein ourselves in on New Year's Eve in order to enjoy a ten or sometimes twelve-hour lunch session somewhere ridiculously fancy without nursing epic hangovers.

Our New Year's Day lunch allowed us to avoid crazy Uber surge prices, overpriced dinner and drinks packages, and the huge crowds that overtook the Sydney waterfront on the year's most popular night out.

'Who's ready for a party?' Nick exclaimed, skipping excitedly around the flimsy blue pool we'd erected on the lawn outside our kitchen.

He was sporting a pair of snug black Speedos and a red, glittery novelty top hat.

'You going to wear that to lunch, mate?' Angus said, raising an eyebrow. 'I think Wild Boys Afloat's going to want its gear back.' We all burst out laughing.

The previous year had been intense, but also extremely rewarding. Eight years of hard slog had begun to pay off, and I was now juggling roles as a print journalist, Nova radio co-host, showbiz commentator for Channel Nine and an event compere. I could have counted on one hand the number of weekends I'd had off during 2015, with most Sunday mornings spent at Nine's Willoughby studios, before heading to Nova to record 'Confidential On Nova', the national radio show I hosted with my long-time colleague and friend, Jonathon 'J.Mo' Moran.

I'd also just turned 30 and was looking forward to this next decade—one that I hoped would be calmer and punctuated by a couple of chubby-cheeked babies.

My 'dirty thirty' had been celebrated with a ten-day Indonesian getaway with Nick, Briana, Mike and Chrissy, and a few other of my closest friends. After a twelve-hour voyage, which had included a flight to Denpasar, a three-hour taxi ride and a perilous fast boat ride from Bali's east coast, we arrived on Gili Trawangan, a tiny island off Lombok known for its pristine beaches and vibrant nightlife.

The Gili Islands were how I imagined Bali would have been decades ago, before the explosion of Bintang-loving Aussie tourists turned a surfing paradise into Indonesia's equivalent of Surfers Paradise.

There was no collective sewerage system on Gili Trawangan, rickety fishing boats delivered the island's fresh water supply daily, and one single dirt road connected the entire island. There were only three modes of transport on Gili—horse and cart, bicycle, and by foot. It was bliss.

The morning after we arrived, my girlfriends and I secured our sun beds around the small pool of the boutique hotel we'd booked for the week. We'd already sized up the pool situation as we'd wheeled our bags to our small, white rooms, calculating there were significantly more hotel guests than lounges. 'Let's meet at the pool by seven,' I said conspiratorially before we'd retired to our rooms. 'You take the Brazilians' spots, and I'll secure the beds the German blokes were on.' We took our holiday relaxation very seriously.

All three of us had fallen ill with colds before we left Sydney, Chrissy and I battling throat and ear infections. But a course of antibiotics, combined with the heat and slow holiday pace, was making me feel a little more human.

'Cheers to the last hurrah!' I said to the girls a few hours into our inaugural pool session, raising a wooden tiki cup in the air. It was filled with ice and a frothy golden liquid, which may have contained a few cheeky nips of white rum and Malibu. I wasn't going to let a little strep throat spoil my party.

We had promised each other we would only check our work emails once a day, which just 24 hours into the trip was already tough. But we needed a break from screens.

The three of us had each achieved many of the goals we had set ourselves at the start of our respective careers. Chrissy had co-founded a successful public relations company and Briana, like myself, worked at *The Daily Telegraph* and had recently joined its Sydney Confidential team. We were all a similar age, and thinking about starting families in the near future.

'We *have* to come back next year,' Chrissy sighed as she sat on the edge of the small pool, her evenly tanned legs lazily churning the water.

'You never know, some of us might have to bring prams,' I mused.

Both girls looked at me curiously, scanning my soft, tanned belly.

'God no!' I exclaimed. 'Not yet. You've just seen me drink two piña coladas!' A smile escaped my lips. 'But seriously, I don't know how prams will go on the island's dirt road—it's totally buggered-up my suitcase wheels.'

◆ ◆ ◆

My role as a fashion and entertainment writer at News Corp had dominated my twenties. I'd stood behind the velvet rope of hundreds of red carpets, interviewed scores of international celebrities and critiqued countless fashion shows. I had covered the rise of hotshot designers and others' falls from grace, been threatened with legal action, and slagged-off on social media by more than a few online trolls.

I still enjoyed my work in the fast-paced world of showbiz reporting, but after almost a decade covering the goings-on of Sydney's social and fashion set, I was exhausted and restless. I was chronically stressed, and in recent years had begun self-medicating with a post-work glass of shiraz. Sometimes it was two glasses; often a whole bottle.

It seemed absurd that I was always so anxious, considering much of my job involved asking Rachael Finch what style hat she'd be wearing to the Melbourne Cup Carnival, and writing stories on why 'red was the new black' for summer swimwear. 'We're not curing cancer,' my colleagues and I would remind each other if we were having a collectively shit day.

But it was intense, and the initial achievement I had felt climbing my way up from coffee-fetcher to covering the most-read pages of the country's top-selling newspaper had waned. I was longing for a new challenge—something that could offer more satisfaction than securing another page-three exclusive detailing Miranda Kerr's new lingerie/beauty/miso soup contract.

Life was far from awful, however. I knew I was lucky to have a job at all, least of all in the media. I had a husband who adored me, and I him; I was healthy and I had a wonderful family, including an arrogant, disdainful and extremely cute cat named Chairman Meow.

In fact, from the outside, things looked pretty darn enviable. Anyone who stalked my Instagram account would have come across selfies with Kim Kardashian, runway photos from the front rows of Fashion Week, group shots of long lunches and the inevitable cat video. But as many of us now realise, the stylised lives we portray on social media are far from the reality.

As grateful as I tried to be for my blessed life, I had begun to want more than tickets to premieres and the buzz of breaking big celebrity news stories. Something deeper, more meaningful.

And so, a month after my 30th birthday, I enrolled in an oil painting class at Sydney Community College. As a kid I loved to draw, so perhaps setting a weekly play date with myself could be just the thing I needed to unleash my creativity and get me out of my motivational slump.

It soon became my favourite day of the week. Every Tuesday I'd slip out of the News Corp building at 5.15 p.m., hoping nobody would see me leaving on time, toting a giant orange Tilly's Art Supplies shopping bag, containing an A3 pad of canvas paper, a dozen small metal tubes of oil paints, paint-brushes of various sizes and a handful of paint-splattered rags. I'd walk up the creaky steps of the former St Joseph's Catholic School in Rozelle, past the small classrooms of old and young Community College students in the midst of sketching portraits and assembling floral bouquets, and into our art studio. I'd drag an old rickety easel from the back wall to my spot in the class, pull out my painting pad and feel the tension in my mind and body relax as I put my crimson or cadmium-soaked brush to the canvas.

The two-hour lesson would fly by, as my eyes flicked between the carefully placed subject matter—usually a combination of crockery items and fruit—and my canvas. It wasn't long before I was hooked. I started painting whenever I had a spare moment, filling up my workbook with fruit and vegetable still lifes and portraits of African animals. Our small inner-west apartment took on a permanent odour of turpentine as my collection of paintings and works-in-progress piled up in the corner.

Art was the outlet I'd been craving. It was meditative. I could spend hours building up details on a patch of fur, or sketch-ing the dimpled peel of an orange, and it would feel like only minutes had passed, my mind having switched from 'monkey' to 'monk' mode. It had helped me sleep better, and I'd become more focused at work.

Maybe a few months maternity leave would be a good chance to flex my artistic muscles . . .

♦ ♦ ♦

Nick interrupted my thoughts as he jumped in the paddle pool, sending bucketfuls of water over its sagging edge and knocking off his novelty top hat, which began to sink as the cardboard millinery absorbed the water.

I dunked my head beneath the fresh, cool liquid of the shallow pool. It was a New Year's baptism, washing away the sins of the past night, of the past year.

I was cleansed, refreshed and ready to take on 2016.

D-Day

28 April 2016

I've always had a profound respect for words. In my career as a journalist I've seen politicians, billionaires and Aussie heroes brought to their knees with just a handful of prepositions, nouns and verbs.

Words have power.

I truly came to realise this on Thursday 28 April, 2016, when a single word tore my world apart.

The day had started innocently enough. I took the M50

express bus from my home in Drummoyne to News Corp in Surry Hills.

I loved my bus commute in the mornings—when I managed to get a seat. I had just started an online nutrition course, and was thoroughly enjoying being a student again. My morning bus rides gave me the chance to read my material and listen to podcasts before my day became a chaotic mess of deadlines, interviews and lodging photo bookings. While I didn't think I wanted to become a natural health practitioner, I really liked the idea of learning something totally unrelated to my profession, and thought it would offer an insight into how to be as healthy as possible before Nick and I got down to the business of starting a family.

Nick often joked that I was the queen of projects. At least twice a year, I would develop an obsession. Generally, these were of the culinary or craft kind. Nick got a taste of this early in our relationship. Shortly after I moved in with him and his flatmate, Berg, in Bondi, I decided to become a raw foodist. I bought a dehydrator, and more than once tried to convince Nick that raw walnut taco 'mince' was as good as the real thing. The pantry, which contained bachelor essentials like salt, pepper, warm beers and microwaveable packet pastas when I moved in, soon filled with jars of maca powder, spirulina and every type of nut imaginable. Looking back, I was well ahead of the trend, as raw food is a huge thing now, and while I still love eating fresh, uncooked produce, my complete dedication to the movement only lasted about nine months. Nick was right, cooked taco mince was much better.

Dumplings, homemade sourdough and bone broths were also among my short-lived passions, plus candle making, floral wreath design, edible gardens and sewing. 'When are you going to have a French cooking phase?' Nick would always ask after I pitched him my latest project.

I realise now that some of my earlier food obsessions stemmed from a lack of body confidence. Like many young women, I never thought I was thin enough, and had convinced myself that eternal happiness was only a five-kilo weight loss away. Fortunately as I grew older, and a little more appreciative of my tall, size 12 figure, my interest in food had shifted from the diets which would make me lose weight, to the way of eating which would make me the healthiest person, and mother, I eventually hoped to become.

I had no idea that in 2016 a single phone conversation, less than an hour into my work day, would force me to take on an entirely new project—one my life would depend on.

I was sitting at my desk with my takeaway flat white, after flicking through the day's papers, and reached into my bag to get my phone. It was about 9.15 a.m., and already I had a missed call. It was from the Royal Prince Alfred's haematology department.

I wasn't supposed to hear back from them for three weeks, once my doctor had received the results from some blood tests I'd had taken the day before.

'Ms Halliwell, we've got your test results sooner than anticipated, and an appointment has been made available for you first thing Monday morning,' the receptionist said when I called the number back. 'We're going to need you to come in, and please bring a family member or loved one with you.'

A loved one? People aren't told to visit the doctor with a significant other unless it's expected they'll be in too much shock or distress to make their own way home.

As I hung up the phone, I'd suddenly lost the ability to breathe. I knew I wouldn't be facing a 'Pop a pill and it'll go away' type of problem when Monday rolled around.

My colleague, Sally, saw the panic in my eyes and came over to my desk. 'Are you okay, babe?' she asked.

My hands were shaking uncontrollably and tears had begun tumbling down my cheeks. 'I'm so scared,' I managed to whisper through hyperventilating sobs. Sally gave me a hug, offering to get me a glass of water. 'Maybe we should order you a cab and get you home,' she added, seeing my distress building.

My reaction would not have been so acute if a relative hadn't received a very similar phone call just a few weeks beforehand. My brother-in-law Angus's dad, Harvey, had been told to see his doctor urgently a few days before the Easter break, and to bring his wife Melanie. Sensing some possibly devastating news, Melanie had told the doctors they would enjoy the long weekend with their three sons and their families before finding out what was wrong. The following week he was diagnosed with terminal cancer.

Sally took me downstairs and put me in a cab, giving the driver my address. On the way home I called Nick, and hearing his voice set me off again. For the first few moments of that call, the only sounds that came out of my mouth were short breaths followed by fresh sobs.

'What's wrong, Elle?' Nick shouted. 'What's happened, are you ok? Where are you?'

'I think I'm really sick,' I managed to say. 'The doctor wants us both to come in on Monday. They got my tests back already and I'm so scared. I wish I didn't have to wait all weekend to find out what's wrong with me.'

Fortunately Nick was self-employed at the time and worked from home, so he was waiting at the front door when my taxi pulled up in front of our house. As soon as I saw him I started to cry again, and he gave me a long hug. When, after a few moments, I managed to calm down, he told me he had called our GP, Don 'Doc' Munro, who is also one of our close friends, to see if he could find out what was going on.

Worst-case scenarios ran through my head as I lay on the couch, waiting for Doc to call back. *Did I have a weird virus? Was it cancer? Was it actually nothing to worry about—just a poorly executed phone call from a new receptionist? Maybe they'd mixed up my test with someone who was actually sick? Yes, that's it—things like that happen all the time at hospitals*, I thought, desperately trying to calm my overactive mind. I'm a hypochondriac at the best of times, so this situation wasn't helping my anxiety levels.

Time slowed down to an excruciating pace as I waited for Doc to call back. Part of me wanted to start Googling *high platelets*, but I couldn't drag myself to my computer, too fearful of what I would find.

◆ ◆ ◆

I'd already done a quick online search two months earlier, after a blood test had indicated an abnormally high level of platelets—the element in blood that causes it to clot. Having too many platelets can put you at risk of deep vein thrombosis or stroke.

My husband and I had been thinking about starting a family, and my girlfriend Briana had suggested I get some blood tests before visiting a naturopath she'd started seeing. Briana, like me, was also interested in nutrition and believed there was a strong link between the mind, body and spirit when it came to all-round good health.

We sat next to each other at *The Daily Telegraph* and would distract each other incessantly with new studies we had found on fertility-boosting foods and what supplements were best for our skin or gut health. We loved showbiz and entertainment, but tended to get more excited about the opening of a new organic cafe near our office than interviewing Hollywood superstars.

Briana had been feeling very low on energy earlier in the year, and it was her naturopath who discovered she was low in zinc. I had been feeling particularly stressed and a bit tired too, so was planning to make an appointment—if I could find time in my ridiculously crammed schedule. I'm all for conventional medicine, but wanted a more holistic opinion on how I could keep my stress levels in check and prime my body for baby-making. I considered discussing it with Doc, but decided there was simply no way the straight-talking GP would be able to advise me on herbal tinctures and alternative therapies.

Briana's naturopath requested her clients have their blood tested to check for any trace mineral deficiencies, so I thought having these results at my first visit would speed up the consulting process. In any case I was curious to know what my folate and vitamin D levels were; platelets were the last thing on my mind.

Doc assured me my elevated platelets were probably nothing serious—most likely just my body reacting to a recent stomach bug that had brought me to see him. I'd fallen ill after a dinner at a French restaurant a few nights prior, and needed a doctor's certificate.

'Come back in two weeks and we'll test you again to make sure they've gone back to a normal level,' he said. I wasn't really paying much attention at the time. I was just happy my folate, iron and vitamin D were in the normal range.

A few weeks later, the evening after I'd had the second blood test done, I was out at dinner with Doc and a few other friends at a Potts Point restaurant.

'I got your results,' Doc told me towards the end of the meal. 'Your platelets are still high—they're actually higher than in the last test.'

My stomach flipped. 'So what does that mean? Should I be worried?' I asked hurriedly.

'No, I wouldn't worry,' he said. 'There's something called essential thrombocythemia, which is when your bone marrow makes too many platelets, but it's manageable. I know a haematologist at the Royal Prince Alfred and I've got a referral for you, just to rule out anything else, but don't stress.'

I was glad at this point we'd finished our mains, as my appetite had disappeared.

When I got home I typed *high platelet levels* into Google. I clicked on a site, which mentioned thrombocythemia. My eyes immediately zoned in on a particular sentence: *Sometimes high platelets can indicate the first sign of cancer.*

Cancer. I suddenly felt light-headed. My cousin had passed away from breast cancer only a few months before, after a hard-fought 19-year battle. She was 42 years old. Natalie had been so brave and strong, dealing with the debilitating illness for such a long time while raising two kids, and, in her final months, being dragged through a messy divorce.

Her life had been cut devastatingly short, and the pain of losing her was still so raw among our family.

Could I be next?

It was hard not to imagine the worst—but further down the article I found some reassurance, managing to almost convince myself I was overreacting. *Some conditions can lead to a high platelet count, such as short-term infection or inflammation*, the article read.

As Doc said, my high platelet count was probably just a response to my stomach bug. Nevertheless, my plan to visit Briana's naturopath suddenly dropped to the bottom of my priority list.

My appointment with the haematology department at Camperdown's Royal Price Alfred Hospital was five weeks away, so there was no point losing sleep over it. With Australian Fashion Week approaching I had a lot of work to do, and I also wanted to get stuck into my nutrition course.

◆ ◆ ◆

It was approaching sunset when Nick got a call from Doc.

'Mate,' Doc said, 'I'm going to come around in a few hours, once I've finished work. They're going to call me back soon to tell me what's going on.'

By this stage I'd calmed myself down with a glass of red wine and was mindlessly watching a *Seinfeld* episode, the one in which George starts eating a Snickers bar with a knife and fork.

It was about 7 p.m. when Doc buzzed at our door. He was, as usual, wearing a T-shirt, jeans, boots and a leather biker jacket, all black. Doc is anything but your average GP. We first met him at a friend's birthday lunch in Cockle Bay more than a decade before, shortly after Nick and I began dating, and I must admit I was initially a little intimidated by him. He was sporting jet-black hair, down to his shoulder blades, and what

I would come to know as his signature all-black ensemble. He would've blended in much better at a Comanchero meet than at a stiff, white-coated medical convention. We didn't really get to talk properly, but when we met again a few years later, Doc and his girlfriend Mora soon became our dearest friends. Since then we have enjoyed countless dinners and in 2008 spent two weeks travelling together in Europe.

It's funny how quickly we put people into neat little boxes of assumptions and stereotypes before we even say 'hello', and Doc was the perfect lesson in why it's never a good idea to judge a book by its cover. He has a sick, very dry sense of humour, but is one of the most intelligent, generous and kindest people you could ever meet. Little did I know that a few years later he would also save my life.

Doc is far from a bleeding heart, but I know that when he sat us down on our couch that night and told us I had a rare form of leukaemia, it was one of the toughest diagnoses he had ever had to give.

I can't really remember much of what Doc said after uttering that awful word, *leukaemia*. A black shadow crowded out my vision until it felt as though I was watching him from inside a long, lightless tunnel. I could hear muffled speech, but the words didn't make sense.

Suddenly an image of my future self appeared in my mind: I was a pale mass of bones covered in a blanket of gossamer-thin, hairless flesh, lying in a hospital bed. I wanted Doc to leave, so I could fall apart in private. I wasn't crying; I was trying to stay composed. We had a guest over, after all. I can't believe I was worrying about social etiquette, but in hindsight it was the perfect distraction from the incomprehensible idea I was dying, as he ran through what I could expect as they found out more about my illness.

Chronic myeloid leukaemia.

That was the type of cancer I had; a slowly progressing cancer of the blood and bone marrow.

'If you're going to get leukaemia, it's one of the better types to have,' Doc said, trying to ameliorate the situation.

If I needed anything to cope with the shock, he explained, he could write me a prescription for alprazolam, aka Xanax. Then he got up, said goodbye, and left.

Nick was the first to break. It was soul-crushing to see my strong, eternally positive husband falling apart before my eyes, wailing as tears poured down his face. 'Not my beautiful girl, why her?' Nick began shouting, over and over again as we held each other. I don't know who he was directing the question to. The universe? God, perhaps? A moment later I too was shaking and sobbing uncontrollably, burying my head in his shoulder. We stayed there for what seemed like hours, just holding each other and letting the diagnosis sink in. I couldn't see a future anymore. Those grand plans of having a family and starting a new chapter together had vanished. My life had instantly been sucked into a vast, cancerous black hole.

I'd called my mum, Carrol, earlier that day to tell her about the call from the haematologist's office, and promised to let her know if we managed to get more information before our appointment on Monday.

But now I didn't want to call her. Mum lived in Brisbane, alone, and would be beyond devastated at the thought of not being close by to comfort me.

'Mum?' I whispered when she picked up the phone.

'What's wrong, Elle? Did you find anything else out?' she asked quickly, the urgency creeping into her voice. It took me a few moments to get my voice to work.

'I've got leukaemia,' I finally managed to say. The words felt thick and foreign on my tongue, like I was reading a script for the first time.

My identity had been ripped away in the space of a few seconds, and I hadn't caught up to this new one that had been thrust upon me. Physically I felt no different to the day before, but according to a blood test, this 'new me' was sick, and cancerous. I couldn't say much more to Mum, but told her I'd know more on Monday.

'It's going to be ok,' I said. I didn't believe my own lie, and I doubt Mum did either. 'I love you so much.'

I hung up the phone before she could respond.

◆ ◆ ◆

The next day was spent trying to come to terms with the diagnosis. I'd gone to see Doc again to take him up on his Xanax offer, as my anxiety had become unbearable overnight. I felt as if a huge anvil was strapped to my chest, and my hands had developed an uncontrollable, sweaty tremor.

I tipped a couple of the little blue pills into my hand. The script advised one pill per day when needed. Instead, I visualised the label as reading *Take as many pills as you like when diagnosed with incurable blood cancer* and downed two.

I floated for a few hours, as Nick dealt with the depressing task of breaking the news to our immediate families and close friends.

On Saturday, two days after what I now refer to as D-Day—Diagnosis Day—I was lying on the couch barely able to move. I was exhausted and physically numb, but my mind was in overdrive. Perhaps it was the mild fascination I had developed for *Doomsday Preppers*, a reality show about people preparing for apocalypses and alien invasions by hoarding canned baked beans and water sterilisation tablets in makeshift bunkers, but I couldn't stop recreating various scenarios in my head about my death, and what I would need to do when that time neared. I'd need a will drafted, I decided, and I'd have to write out a list to divvy up my designer shoes amongst my girlfriends. Unfortunately my sisters' feet were too small, so they would get my handbags and jewellery.

My thoughts suddenly returned to a day in late August the previous year, when I visited my accountant to file my tax return. 'You should really consider getting income and life insurance,' he told me. 'If anything happened to you or your husband and you couldn't work, you would need to consider how you'd pay the rent, bills . . . things like that.'

I'd actually asked a financial planner about it afterwards, and decided that my superannuation fund had something similar enough, which would do—because why would I pay several grand a year for something that we wouldn't need to worry about until we were in our sixties? Nick and I were young, fit and invincible. Nothing could happen to us, so it'd be a complete waste of money.

Idiot.

Between these morbid thoughts, I tried to sleep. Maybe, I surmised, if I kept sleeping, I'd eventually wake up from this nightmare. I was still in complete disbelief about my cancer. It didn't seem possible. I felt as healthy as I had ever been, and I couldn't remember the last time I'd taken a sick day. My energy levels fluctuated a bit and I'd had anxiety for years, but I put that down to my job, working long hours and the stresses of deadlines.

Why couldn't I have gotten breast cancer, or some kind of malignant lump, I wondered over and over again. At least I could see it on an ultrasound, or feel it with my hand. Instead, my leukaemia was like a phantom, an invisible entity I simply had to believe existed, based on a few numbers printed on an A4 piece of paper. To me, my blood cancer was nothing bar a numbered cell in an Excel spreadsheet.

I couldn't just get it cut out, removed with a scalpel, and have the hole sewn up nice and neatly. It was in my veins, my bones, my very DNA. I *was* cancer, and cancer was me.

Nick and I were pretending to watch a movie that afternoon, both of us silently contemplating my bleak future as we stared at the TV. 'Those first few days were like a nightmare,' Nick recalled a few months later. 'I'd wake up each morning and for a moment think it had all just been a horrible dream, and then realise it wasn't.' I'd never seen my husband, whose default mental state is positive and happy, look so beaten. He hadn't shaved, and all of his work commitments had been put on hold. I started thinking about our dream of starting a family later that year. We hadn't exactly been careful with contraception, but I had taken a pregnancy test two weeks prior that had come back negative.

Nick had been just as excited as me about having a baby in the not-too-distant future. We'd travelled, partied and done all of the things any newly married couple should have done before parenthood. But my diagnosis had ripped this away from him. If I did survive this disease, neither of us knew whether my fertility would be affected or not.

I'll never know what prompted me to take the spare Clearblue test sitting on top of the fridge on that Saturday afternoon. I actually forgot to check it after I'd gone to the toilet and peed on the little stick. I'd been distracted by something on the TV and had left it on the coffee table while it developed. It was about an hour later that I finally remembered to check it.

It took my brain a moment to catch up to my eyes when I looked at the small display panel on the plastic stick. I was reading it but struggled to comprehend the two words and two numbers it showed, despite their clear, bold font.

Pregnant. 3–4 weeks it read.

Fuck.

Oh, Baby

30 April 2016

I flung the test away, flinching as if it was a piping-hot metal rod.

It skidded across the coffee table towards Nick, who was half-asleep and sprawled on the couch opposite.

I hadn't thought things could get much worse, but seeing that positive test made me realise the battle I faced had just become much more complicated. I hadn't even come to terms with the fact my own life was in danger, but now there were two lives at stake. I felt bile rising up my throat.

The sound of the test hitting the coffee table jolted Nick out of his reverie, and a look of realisation crossed his face when he saw what I'd thrown. He didn't know I'd taken the test, so it took him a while to react as he read and re-read the tiny text on the stick.

'We're going to have a *baby!*' he gasped.

I looked at him, puzzled. 'Are you kidding me?' I hissed, with more anger than I had intended. Nick had always been the more positive person in the relationship, but his reaction to this news was just insane.

Did he not realise what this meant? How complicated this made things?

'How can you possibly think this is good news!?' I exclaimed. 'I've got bloody cancer; I could be dying, so this is far from an ideal situation, Nick!'

Nick, unbeknownst to me, had been doing some Googling on chronic myeloid leukaemia and found a YouTube video featuring a doctor in the UK named Jane Apperley. In the video Professor Apperley mentioned that in Britain, a number of women diagnosed with CML during pregnancy had been treated with alternative medications to the standard oral drugs until the birth of their baby.

There was no mention how far along in their pregnancy they were, or how advanced their cancer was, but it was a thread of hope for Nick to hold onto, and he wasn't letting go.

At my initial visit to the haematologist, the day before my diagnosis, I had mentioned that we were considering trying for a baby later in the year.

'Look, I think it's best you hold off until we get the results back from the blood tests,' he counselled. At the time, I hadn't thought anything of his comment, but he must have sensed something was wrong, despite my lack of obvious symptoms. He had asked me if I'd had any bruising, unexplained weight loss or stomach pains in the last few months.

'I had gastro a few weeks ago, but that's about it,' I replied. Suddenly I remembered something that could have been a symptom. 'Actually, last week I got a weird sensation in my eyes. They went kind of blurry, like a kaleidoscope, but it only lasted a couple of minutes. I thought maybe I'd been looking at the computer for too long at work.'

The haematologist scribbled it all down in my file, then sent me downstairs to the pathology centre to have some blood taken. I blanched when I saw the nurse walk in juggling a dozen empty vials.

'Are they all for me?' I asked, my mouth opening in shock. I'd never had more than three samples taken at one time, and immediately regretted having skipped lunch in favour of a strong flat white.

'They sure are,' the nurse chuckled. She was a large woman, of Islander appearance, and had a reassuring demeanour.

'Is this the most you've ever had to take in one go?' I asked, trying to distract myself from the needle as it broke through the flesh of my forearm.

'I think my record is fifteen, so you're pretty close,' she said, smiling warmly.

I called Nick as I left the pathology centre. The sheer number of blood vials I'd had to fill had made me feel light-headed, and I started to wonder what exactly the haematologist was looking for. Nick asked how everything went, and after explaining what the haematologist had said about us holding off trying for a baby, my eyes started to pool with tears. 'What if it's not *nothing*?' I asked Nick. 'What if there is seriously something wrong with me?'

'Elle, take it easy,' Nick said. Having lived with me for the best part of a decade, he knew I had a tendency to be a catastrophist, and could calm me down with just a few strategic words. 'There's nothing to worry about. And if there is—which there won't be—there's no point stressing about it now.'

'You're right,' I said. I took a tissue from my bag and dabbed the corners of my eyes, trying to avoid ruining my makeup. I had a showbiz report for Channel Nine's afternoon news to do in an hour, and didn't have time to re-do my whole face.

I had no idea at the time that the haematologist's advice on holding off our baby plans had come much too late—and that an embryo the size of a sesame seed was already growing inside me.

I was only a few days into parenthood, and already I felt like a bad mother.

Part of me resented this miracle, which had denied me the ability to medicate the reality of my diagnosis away. The hurt and the fear couldn't be drowned away with an $8 bottle of cab sav. I had no choice but to tackle this situation head-on, and completely, unbearably, sober.

There was a bottle of vodka perched on top of our pantry. It had gold flecks floating at the bottom—the promise of riches to whoever downed the last two nips. Would it really matter, I thought to myself as I stared at the clear liquor. I imagined it stinging as it hit the back of my throat, then slowly numbing every part of me.

This baby didn't stand a chance inside a body that was already busy fighting millions of deadly cancer cells, anyway.

How could it support new life as well as trying to keep itself alive? Something would have to give.

I reached for the bottle, its metallic confetti swirling like snow in a snow dome as I carried it slowly into the storeroom.

'I'll come back for you in a few weeks, once this is all over,' I told it, before pushing the clear bottle to the back of the dusty shelf.

◆ ◆ ◆

Nick and I didn't talk much as we drove to the Royal Prince Alfred Hospital on the Monday morning. We had run out of tears, run out of comforting words to tell each other. We were both exhausted from hearing sobs through our mobile phones, and running through the same tragic story over and over and over again.

Today was the day I was supposed to have received my diagnosis. It was only four days, but it felt like an eternity had passed since Doc had said that word, *leukaemia*. The word still felt strange, each syllable a dumbbell that rolled around my mouth. We'd had the whole weekend to prepare for this meeting, and had armed ourselves with an exhaustive list of questions for the haematologist, who we would come to refer to as Prof.

I'd spent all morning doing my makeup and hair, tidying myself up after spending the best part of four days in the same trackpants and the same sweater, the neckline of which had become stiff from absorbing countless salty tears.

If I was going to have to tackle this illness, I wasn't going to do it looking like shit.

I paid more attention as I entered the Chris O'Brien Lifehouse clinic, the RPA's cancer centre, for the second time.

The first time—a week prior when I had been for the initial consultation and undergone the blood tests—I had popped in during my lunch break and barely looked up from my phone, too busy responding to emails to take in details of the building.

Like most people, I hate hospitals. The smell of bleach and the hum and intensity of fluorescent lighting leave me feeling edgy, icky and depressed.

But the three-year-old Lifehouse building didn't give off a sanatorium vibe. It was shiny and modern, almost inviting—a place you wouldn't mind spending time in while waiting to hear news about your cancer.

A woman was knitting woollen beanies at a small craft station as we arrived, a glass display cupboard full of assorted paintings, sculptures and art projects beside her. Across the foyer a cafe selling Campos espresso and fresh sandwiches was operating, its customers a mix of patients and specialists working on their laptops, reading the day's paper and chatting to each other over hot cups of caffeinated liquid.

At first glance, it could have been the foyer of any one of Sydney's CBD office buildings, and that relaxed me. I could imagine I was visiting my accountant, or a bank, rather than my blood cancer specialist.

We took the glass elevator to level two, which housed the centre's clinics, and checked in at reception. I took a brochure to flick through before we sat down on one of the armless beige sofas to wait for our appointment. The pamphlet contained information on the new centre, which opened in 2013. The Lifehouse was the vision of Professor Chris O'Brien, who in 2003 had been appointed the director of the RPA Sydney Cancer

Centre, and was determined to create a world-class centre for treatment and research into the devastating disease.

In a tragic twist, Professor O'Brien was diagnosed with a malignant brain tumour in 2006 and died three years later, just a few months after the centre received the backing of state and federal governments. He never got the chance to walk through the doors of the Lifehouse he had worked so tirelessly to create—a building that would become a haven for those dealing with the illness, and for their loved ones.

The floor below us contained a wellness space called the Living Room, where patients could trial complementary therapies in conjunction with their cancer treatment. It offered yoga, qigong, acupuncture and massage, as well as counselling, and exercise and diet advice. I am a big believer in holistic approaches to health, and was heartened to see alternative treatments given a place alongside modern medicine.

While waiting to see the Prof, I picked up my phone and opened up Instagram. I scrolled through my feed, and my eyes landed upon a quote a friend had posted. I took a screen shot and posted it on my own: *I get so offended when my body decides we're gonna get sick, like, I fed you a vegetable last week, how DARE you betray me like this. Ungrateful. Offended.* A smile threatened to break across my lips. It wasn't quite a grin, but it was the first time my mood had ticked above 'Unbearable' on the emotional chart since D-Day.

'We've found out something since Thursday which could change things,' Nick told Prof after we sat down in his small private clinic room. We didn't want to get caught up in treatment details before giving him the whole picture.

'Elle's pregnant.'

The Prof was the first person we had shared the news with—not our parents, not our sisters, or our closest friends. There would be no hugs, no congratulations, and no questions as to when we were due. That moment, which had filled so many expectant parents with joy for countless generations, would be denied to us.

We knew not to expect a positive response, but the Prof's reaction was a blow to the chest, all the same.

'Shit,' he eventually said.

Hearing that word from the Professor's mouth seemed more awkward than disheartening. He was a quietly spoken man, in his late fifties, whose quiet, serious disposition didn't naturally align itself with words like 'shit'.

Prof had been researching my treatment options since receiving my blood test results. Knowing my desire to have a baby, he had consulted with an expert in Adelaide, Professor Tim Hughes, as to the best way to protect my fertility, and form a contingency plan if my treatment made conception difficult. Professor Hughes, I would later discover, was a world expert in chronic myeloid leukaemia, and at the forefront of research into a cure for the disease. Nick had also come across his name during a Google search over the weekend; Professor Hughes had commented on a forum post regarding a woman who was planning to stop treatment for her leukaemia in order to have a baby.

Our baby news had thrown a very large spanner into the works.

'I've never treated anyone who was pregnant at the time of diagnosis,' Prof admitted. He didn't even *know* of anyone who had been in our situation. We subsequently learnt that even Professor Hughes had not looked after a patient in my situation either.

I had never felt more alone.

'What we were going to discuss, before I knew about the pregnancy, was the possibility of delaying treatment so we could harvest some eggs, see the fertility unit, and get them to fertilise some embryos *in vitro* and freeze them, so you've got that as a backup regardless of what else happens in the future,' Prof explained.

'The problem there, is that it would delay starting these drugs for a bit longer—and the issue we have to think about is the risk that your very early chronic myeloid leukaemia, or CML, might transform and progress to an acute leukaemia.'

Acute leukaemia.

Nick squeezed my hand. A mate of Nick's from high school had been diagnosed with acute leukaemia several years before, and had undergone a bone marrow transplant. Nick had seen first hand the devastating effects blood cancer—and even more so its treatments—could have on the body. And just a few months ago, Nick had learned his mate's leukaemia had returned, and things were not looking good. Tragically, less than a year after celebrating his wedding, he was fighting for his life, once again.

If the Prof believed delaying treatment for even a few months to have my eggs frozen might cause my chronic illness to develop into acute leukaemia, even *considering* keeping the baby seemed ludicrous, I thought.

The new lifesaving drugs that had recently been made available in Australia under the Pharmaceutical Benefits Scheme were not an option during pregnancy. Early studies had shown that if mothers taking tyrosine kinase inhibitors did manage to carry to full term, there was a significant possibility of malformation. The rate of miscarriage and stillbirth was also significantly high.

'We just don't know what could happen, and the last thing you want on top of everything else is a damaged baby,' Prof said, looking apologetic. 'If you were to keep this pregnancy, the only option would be to start you on interferon—but it's not an easy drug to take, compared to the kinase inhibitors.'

'Do you mean in terms of side effects?' Nick asked.

The Prof nodded. Severe nausea, body aches, fever, hallucinations and depression were just a few of the side effects linked to interferon, a drug commonly administered to people with AIDS, hepatitis or multiple sclerosis.

Interferons are naturally occurring proteins in the body that respond to and alert the immune system to the presence of pathogens, and while the drug had been used to treat chronic myeloid leukaemia prior to the discovery of tyrosine kinase inhibitors, in terms of long-lasting effectiveness it was a very inferior alternative.

'Interferon is not the best by a long way,' Prof explained. 'There was a trial called IRIS, which was the first trial of imatinib—the first kinase inhibitor—against the best available therapy at that time, which was a combination of interferon and a chemo drug called cytarabine. The results for imatinib were vastly superior to those for interferon.

'If you had a disease that was very well controlled, but not completely negative, and wanted to *then* get pregnant—*then* you could make a reasonable case for switching to interferon. But to rely on interferon to induce control of your leukaemia during pregnancy? I don't think it's a good idea.' His reasons for that statement were based on several concerns. First, I might not be able to tolerate interferon well during pregnancy. Second, not only was interferon and cytarabine clearly inferior to kinase inhibitor treatment, I would have to use interferon by itself as cytarabine could definitely not be used during the first part of my pregnancy.

One of the questions that had continued to cross my mind was whether or not this baby could end up with leukaemia. If there was a strong chance the baby could inherit this dreaded disease, then it would certainly sway my decision towards termination. I couldn't bear the thought of having to watch a loved one deal with this dreadful disease, let alone my own child.

Prof shook his head. 'The baby would have the same chance as anyone of getting CML,' he said. 'It's genetic, but it's not hereditary, so it can't be passed on.'

Prof booked me in for a bone marrow biopsy, for the following week. He also suggested we arrange an appointment with one of the hospital's fertility specialists to discuss my options in the event we chose to terminate the pregnancy.

He called the fertility centre while we waited, to book me in. 'We saw her only a week ago for thrombocytosis, but it turns out to be CML,' he said to the woman on the other end of the line. It was strange hearing him discuss my illness in front of me, with a person I had never met. I felt disconnected.

'She mentioned then she was hoping to get pregnant, and we were talking about how we would organise eggs and things like that—but when she's come in today to make some plans, it turns out she's already pregnant, which complicates our initial management. I think she still needs to see you to discuss pregnancies and options, because we may recommend a termination at this stage.

'Ideally we would start the kinase inhibitors in a couple of weeks. We could delay, but the risks start to go up the longer we delay.'

He hung up the phone, and turned to us.

Prof understood our dilemma. He agreed the idea of terminating a pregnancy in order to ensure my future fertility seemed counterintuitive. Ethically, it seemed to me like a pretty fucked-up thing to do. But I was seriously considering it, nevertheless. It would give me a better chance of survival—and the best odds of being able to start a family down the track— than the alternative choices.

But at the end of the day *I* was Prof's patient, not my unborn child, and my health and survival was, and had to be, his main priority. He couldn't force me to choose one option over another; all he could do was offer me choices and his professional advice on the safest route for me to take.

'There's a lot to discuss about side effects, but we still have to focus on this pregnancy issue,' Prof said.

'I'll be brutal,' he added. 'The best is if there is no pregnancy now. But it's your choice.'

'Would you be okay if we got in touch with Professor Hughes?' Nick asked. 'If he's a CML expert, he might have some extra info for us.'

'Sure,' said Prof, scribbling notes in my thin, beige-coloured medical file.

♦ ♦ ♦

There was too much to take in. I felt incredibly drained as we left the Lifehouse and drove home.

I didn't have the energy to talk to Nick about what had just transpired, so I just stared out the window as the car drove along Parramatta Road, distracting myself with the movements of pedestrians going about their day. I wanted Nick to keep driving.

To drive me far away from this complicated mess. I dreaded the cessation of the engine and the deafening silence, which would force me to contemplate the impossible choice I now faced.

I had, in a way, started to come to terms with my cancer diagnosis and, pregnancy aside, what it could mean for me in the future. From the information Nick had found online and our meeting with Prof, I had begun to get a fairly good idea of the disease I was facing.

First of all, cancer sucks. But not all cancers are created equal, so it was with this in mind that I attempted to work through the cons and pros of my diagnosis to get a clearer picture of my illness.

The biggest con was that it was cancer. Nobody wants to get cancer, especially when they're 30 years old and busy with much more exciting stuff like 30th birthday parties and making babies. Another downside was it is incurable. Yep, nothing bar a very risky bone marrow transplant would give me any hope of ridding myself of this illness, and according to Prof it wasn't even an option worth discussing just yet.

On the upside, I wouldn't have to have surgery to get it removed, as it was literally in my bones and blood. *Come to think of it, that's another con,* I decided.

CML was also quite rare, accounting for just 0.03 per cent of all cancers diagnosed in Australia. Definitely a con, as rare cancers often get overlooked when it comes to research and awareness.

It was, however, a slow-growing cancer, which was a pro, especially in my current situation. I wasn't going to wake up the next day and be read my last rites. It could take years for it to kill me, if I wasn't treated, as it progressed in three stages.

The chronic phase could last anywhere from one to three years, and often presented with no symptoms. Over time, immature white blood cells called granulocytes or leukaemic blasts multiplied in the bone marrow and bloodstream, leading to the accelerated phase. At this point patients could expect bruising, anaemia, infections and weight loss before progressing to blast crisis, which in just a few months could become fatal.

Another pro was that in the last fifteen years a new drug had emerged on the market called a tyrosine kinase inhibitor. Until the release of Gleevec, the world's first tyrosine kinase inhibitor, the outlook for CML patients was grim: according to America's National Cancer Institute, fewer than one in three survived five years past diagnosis. Fortunately these new TKI drugs had changed this, and survival rates around the world had improved significantly.

Another con was that the TKI drugs I would eventually need to take came with some pretty nasty side effects. Nausea, skin rashes, hair loss, weakened immunity, fluid retention, liver and heart problems were just a few of the issues I could potentially have to deal with. Fatigue was another major con, and something many patients battled with years after their illness had been brought under control.

For someone who was juggling a TV, radio and television career and a bunch of other hobbies and commitments, would I have to give them all up?

Would I be too tired to enjoy all of the things I loved, and spend my days resting with a knitted blanket over my knees?

Prof had reassured me that many CML survivors went on to live relatively normal lives thanks to these new drugs, if they adhered to the strict dosages prescribed and followed a healthy diet and lifestyle. But fatigue was a common side effect, and it was something I must prepare for.

There were definitely fewer pros than cons, not even taking into account the pregnancy, but compartmentalising them into neat lists gave me a small sense of control over my unknowable future.

◆ ◆ ◆

Unlike my husband, I loathe talking through problems. When I'm confronted with strong emotions, I shut down. My instinct is to run, to remove myself from the situation, and let the problem die away. Sometimes, it disappears. Most of the time, however, it doesn't. It grows, and stretches, until a small crack becomes a chasm that gets harder and harder to fill in. Let enough problems ruminate and you're left with a honeycomb relationship that no amount of Spakfilla can repair.

Nick's perseverance during the early years of our relationship, encouraging me to talk through problems, eventually paid off. Over time, my tendency to detach never quite disappeared, but I became better at communicating my feelings and resolving arguments in the moment, rather than retreating into myself.

As we neared home, Nick turned to me and said, 'I think we should go and see Professor Hughes.'

'In Adelaide?' I asked.

Nick nodded. 'Yeah, let's get a second opinion. If he's a world expert, then he would *have* to have seen a situation like ours before, right?'

I tilted my head thoughtfully. 'Let's think about it,' I said after a moment, then turned back to look out the window.

I still wasn't ready to confront this dilemma. I couldn't shake my belief that the pregnancy wouldn't survive past 12 weeks. And regrettably, in a way, I wanted that to be the case, as it would absolve me of responsibility. I wouldn't feel like a coward knowing I had no choice but to start the lifesaving drugs and protect myself.

I had recently read that about one in five pregnancies ended in miscarriage, with about 80 per cent occurring within the first trimester. The odds of me getting CML were about one in 100,000, I thought—so a one in five chance of losing the baby was statistically very much higher. Considering my body was in crisis, the chance of this pregnancy lasting seemed minuscule.

But the moment I thought about the tiny embryo, this seed of hope germinating in my womb, the idea of losing it was inconceivable.

It had given me a reason to live—a tiny beacon of light flashing in a sea of blackness, urging me to stay afloat and find a safe harbour.

While the Prof had shed more light on my illness at our appointment, Nick and I left with so many more questions.

'If you get onto the chat groups for CML and tell your story, someone else might say, *That's happened to me!*' Prof had suggested. Being a journalist, I was confident my research skills would make it easy for me to track down other women who had faced this same situation. *Someone* down. But it was near impossible. I couldn't find anyone. A precedent was all I wanted. I needed to know how another's story ended, so I could figure out where to go with my own.

I felt so alone.

A Mother's Choice

Dear baby,

My name's Elle, but you can call me 'Mum'. You don't have a name, and I'm not sure if you ever will. I don't know if you'll ever say my name, or look into my eyes as you're falling asleep in my arms.

It's Mother's Day today. Your grandmother is staying with us at the moment, because I'm sick. She wouldn't have been here for it otherwise, so I guess that's one positive thing that's come from last week's crappy news. I know it's not really officially Mother's Day for me, but I doubt I'll have anything to celebrate next year, so I'm going to pretend—just for today—that I'm healthy and have nothing to fear. I don't think we're going to do much today; nobody in the family is really in the mood for champagne and finger sandwiches at the moment.

You only came into my world a few weeks ago, and I'll be frank: your timing was terrible. I don't know why you chose me to give you life of all the millions of potential mothers out there. Sure, I'm a pretty good cook and your grandparents are awesome, but my body's struggling to keep itself alive, let alone you. If you're anything like your dad, though, you don't back down from challenges.

The doctor says the safest choice would be to send you back, to that place we go before and after we're alive. I don't know what it's like there. What I do know is that that place is not here, with me, your mum. How could I send you there when I'm scared of going myself? How could I deny you the joy of feeling snowflakes fall on your nose for the first time, or being tickled with kisses until you can't breathe? I've done all of that. I've played in the mud, travelled to far-off places and been visited by Santa Claus and The Easter Bunny too many times to count.

I saw you in my dreams the other night. You had blue eyes, like your dad; a head of fine, sandy hair and bright red, chubby cheeks.

And I loved you. Whatever happens, know that I wanted you, so, so much and I already adore you.

    All my love,

    Mum

I've always loved photography. The camera—an object that has the ability to capture moments in time—still fascinates me, and I have been almost obsessive about documenting my life through the camera ever since I first got my hands on one. My dad's giant shed contains boxes and boxes of photographs I've taken, capturing friend's birthdays, overseas holidays and random happy snaps. Perhaps it's one of the reasons I became a journalist: that desire to tell a story of a moment in time which can never be relived.

A few days after our visit with Prof, Nick and I had dinner with two of our close friends, Alex and Paul. Nick thought taking me out of the house would help me forget our troubles for a while, and by the time our food arrived, it had worked; I almost felt like myself again. Nick had called them after my diagnosis to break the news, and after a brief chat about how I was feeling, the conversation quickly moved on to topics like politics and the global economy. I tend to prefer less argumentative discussions over dinner, but it was a blissful distraction from my own dramas nevertheless. Alex, who worked in breakfast TV, had an incredibly broad knowledge of current affairs. He also loved sinking his teeth into a good yarn.

'You should keep a video diary of what's going on,' Alex suggested towards the end of our dinner, taking a sip of red wine. 'You know, just as a record.'

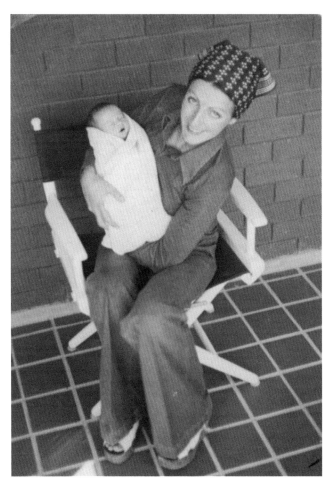

My mum with my late
brother Eric in 1974.

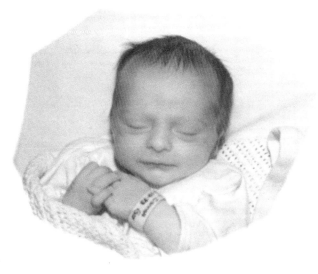

My brother, Eric.

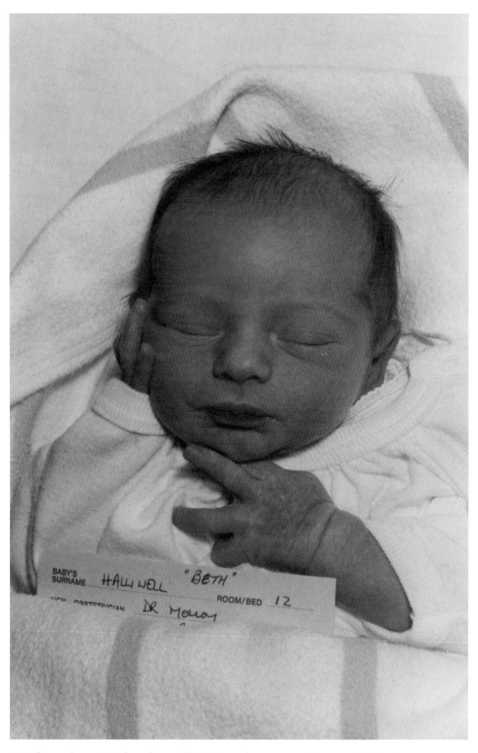

BABY'S SURNAME HALLIWELL "BETH"

ROOM/BED 12

DR Molloy

My first photo. It's hard to tell Eric and me apart in our birth photos.
Mum still thinks I'm him, reincarnated.

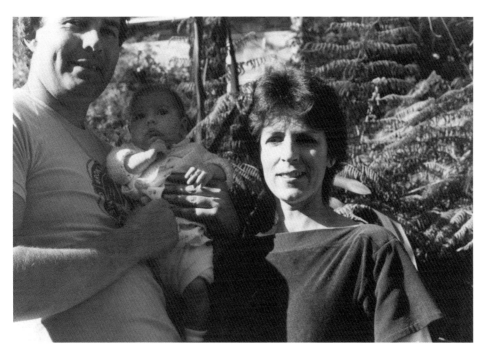

As a baby with my parents, Ross and Carrol.

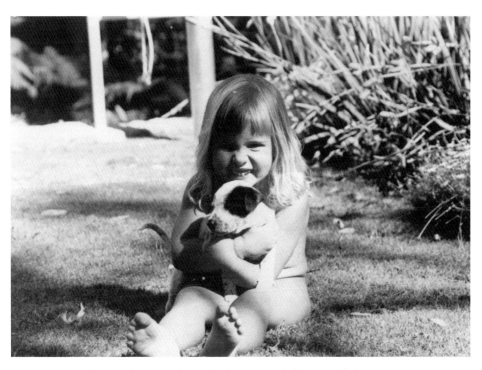

I loved animals much more than clothing until the age of about six. Here I am with my sister Amy's dog, Lani, when I was about three years old.

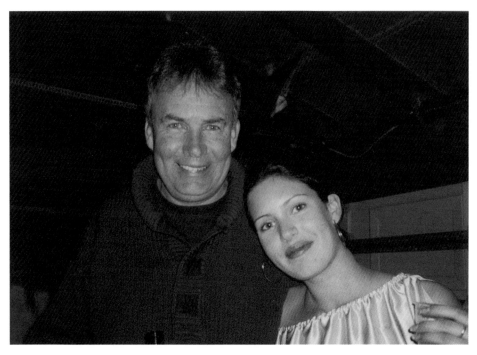

Me and Dad on my sixteenth birthday.

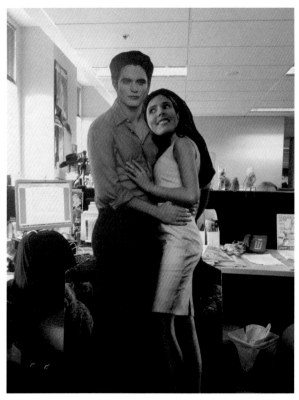

Mucking around with the life-sized Robert Pattinson cut-out beside my desk at the beginning of my R-Patz obsession.

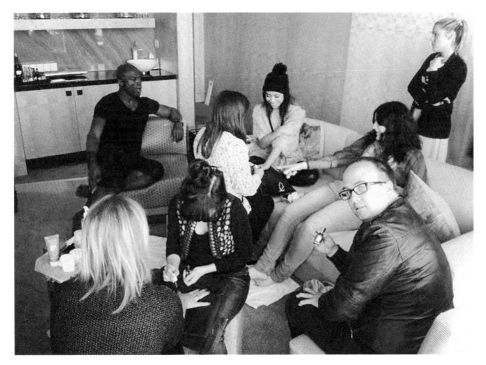

J.Mo and I having mani-pedis with Seal at The Darling Hotel in 2012 during the first season of *The Voice Australia*.

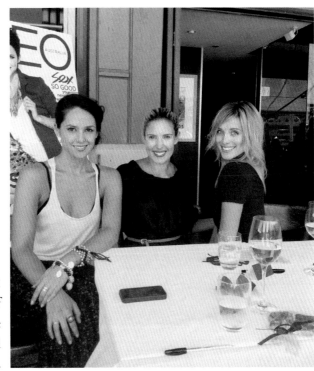

Judging the 2012 Cleo Bachelor of The Year with Zoe Marshall and Casey Burgess.

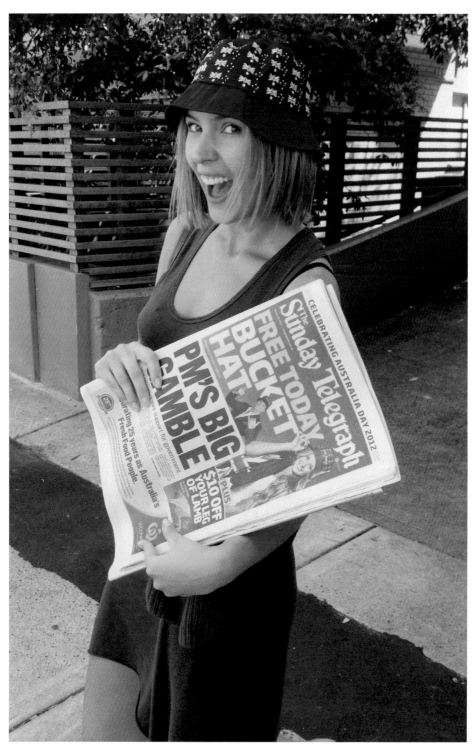

I always did, and still do, love sitting down and reading the paper before work and on the weekend.

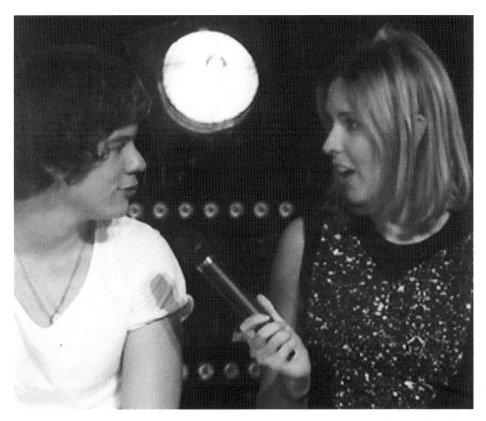

Interviewing Harry Styles during One Direction's promotional trip ahead of their 2013 Take Me Home Tour.

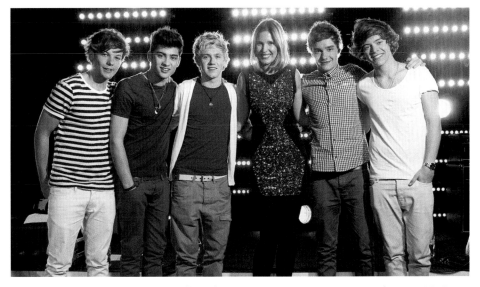

Posing with One Direction after their intimate gig at Fox Studios in 2012. This became the page 3 picture. (© NEWS CORP/ Sam Ruttyn)

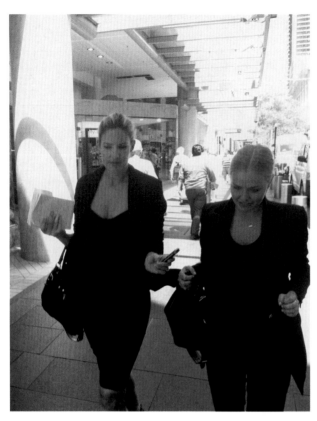

Interviewing Lara Worthington (nee Bingle) in 2013 when she launched her swimwear range for Cotton On Body.

I've interviewed Miranda Kerr a lot, most of which occurred during her time as the face of David Jones. This was taken backstage before the David Jones Autumn/ Winter fashion launch in 2013.

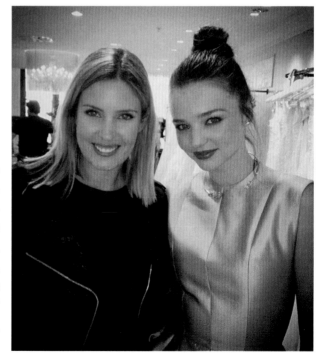

I thought it over for a moment. It was actually a good idea. My mind was so foggy I could barely remember my own phone number at the time, so there was no chance I would be able to keep track mentally of everything that was happening. It would also be a good way to track my symptoms as my disease progressed. And a way to record my pregnancy, in the unlikely event that I gave birth.

Video diary, 5 May 2016

Hi. I don't know who I'm saying 'hi' to, but anyway. I'm still in a lot of shock about what's happened in the past week, but yeah, I've hardly slept, which you can probably tell from the bags under my eyes. So I found out on Thursday that I've got leukaemia and then on Saturday that I'm pregnant. I still don't think it's all sunk in. I feel so weak and exhausted, probably from all the crying and having to tell everyone about the cancer. It couldn't be the pregnancy, I don't think, 'cause I can't be more than a couple of weeks pregnant and I'm pretty sure you don't get any symptoms for a few more weeks. Maybe it's the cancer? Anyway, I still have to get a proper blood test to check I am really pregnant and get an ultrasound, which I can't get for a few more weeks until I'm further along. It's all so overwhelming. We haven't told anyone about the baby yet, because we don't know what we're going to do, and Prof reckons we shouldn't go through with it. I'm so scared about what's going to happen. I'm going to try and do these videos regularly, but we'll see how we go. Anyway, bye.

A Mother's Love

I was lucky to have been born, according to Mum. I was her fourth child and third daughter, and with a gap of nine years between my sister Amy and me, I was a very big surprise to my parents. They were convinced their days of broken sleep and nappy changes were well and truly behind them.

Mum is the most kind, loving woman—but before she had my brother, Eric, she wasn't very interested in kids or babies. She immediately realised after he was born that it was just *other* people's kids she didn't like; she was besotted from the moment she laid eyes on him. He was born twelve years before me, and had olive skin, long limbs like his dad, and a frown on his face, 'as if he were trying to solve a riddle,' Mum said.

One Sunday morning, when Eric was only nine weeks old, Mum's world was shattered.

'I awoke to sunlight shining in through the window, and nudged your dad awake,' she told me. 'I was calculating in my mind the hours since Eric's last feed, and slowly realised something was wrong.' Eric hadn't woken up for his 1 a.m. feed, and hadn't slept this long before, so Dad went to wake him.

'An eternity seemed to pass,' Mum remembered, 'and I dragged myself out of bed.' My dad was standing in the hallway, staring into Eric's room. He didn't look at her or move a muscle. It was like he was glued to the wall.

'Oh, for God's sake, Ross!' Mum said impatiently, walking towards Eric.

'Don't go in there, Carrol!' Dad said. 'He's dead.'

Mum never saw her baby boy ever again.

'I wanted so much to hold him just one more time—and yet I didn't want to see him that way,' she admitted. 'I wanted to pretend it wasn't real. In retrospect, I am glad I didn't go in, because I would rather my last memory was the one of kissing him goodnight.'

My brother had died of sudden infant death syndrome, the coroner later confirmed. I can't even comprehend how hard it would have been for her, and my Dad, to lose their first child, just months after he came into their lives.

Unlike Mum, her own mother—who I call Nana Long—didn't have much of a maternal side. I spent countless weekends as a child with Granny, Dad's mum, but have barely any memories of Nana Long from my youth. Perhaps it was because Mum didn't get along with her, rather than her lack of desire to see the grandchildren. But she rarely called on birthdays or sent cards, and I never really got to know much about her, except from the stories Mum told me about her own childhood.

The oldest of three children, Mum grew up in Sydney's western suburbs in a small, white weatherboard house with her mother. At the age of five, she and her siblings were sent to a children's home in Parramatta, where they stayed for three years.

Mum has often described her childhood as miserable.

'We were lucky to get a visit from our mother once a month,' she said. 'My mother remarried, and eventually we went to live with my stepfather, who was a monster. Not from drink, as he didn't drink—and on the rare occasion he did he was actually a reasonable person. No, he was just a brute of the worst kind.'

My dad's childhood, in contrast, was a pleasant one. Raised in Manly Vale, he was one of six children and spent his child-hood building go-karts, terrorising the neighbourhood with his bicycle gang, the Byfans, and swimming in Manly Dam. 'Our mums would wave us goodbye and tell us not to be home after dark,' Dad recalls fondly. 'We'd usually come back at lunch, because we had no money, but then we'd go back out again until dinner. We used to make canoes out of corrugated iron and planks of wood, which we'd attach on either end, and then we'd tar it up to stop the water coming in, and paddle around the dam. A couple of kids drowned in the dam in those days, because there was just no supervision. We didn't have a lot of money, but me and my brothers and sisters had a lot of fun as kids.'

My parents would never forget the pain of losing Eric, which would follow them through their lives, but the birth of my eldest sister Martine two years later, in 1975, brought back some of the joy they had lost.

Mum believes Martine became a night owl because she was poked and prodded constantly while sleeping to make sure she was breathing. 'I had to remind myself that the chances of my losing another baby to SIDS were extremely remote and to leave the poor kid alone,' Mum admits.

A year and five days later Amy came into the world, and Mum and Dad felt their family was complete.

◆ ◆ ◆

A few years after my sister Amy was born, Mum died.

She was only dead for a few minutes, in the Crown Street Women's Hospital in Sydney, but her heart stopped beating nonetheless. To this day she can still vividly recall having an out-of-body experience, and I often ask her to retell the story, as I have always had a fascination with the afterlife and the mystery of what happens when we die.

'I remember lying on the treatment table, telling the nursing sister I was too tired to "fight the feeling"—and next thing I knew I was sitting on top of a metal locker, with my legs hanging over the side,' Mum explained. 'I looked down and saw a large woman on a stepladder, her arms raised above her head with what looked like a foot in each hand.'

Mum said she somehow drifted closer to the scene, and could see monitors and equipment flashing and a group of people rushing around her lifeless body.

'I heard someone say "She's flat-lined!", and then as I watched I calmly decided that I should get back.'

Mum says she nearly turned around and went the other way, because she felt so peaceful, but thoughts of her family changed her mind.

'It was the most pleasant feeling I have ever had,' Mum said. 'I'm a little disappointed I never got to see angels, or bright lights, or loved ones gone before, but I do know that when you die it isn't entirely over, and that's a comfort.'

Mum's four-minute death was the result of a haemorrhage. She had lost three litres of blood, due to a tear in her womb from the removal of an intrauterine device.

Rather than have a hysterectomy to stop the bleeding, Mum chose to trial an experimental drug, which fortunately got her back on her feet.

◆ ◆ ◆

In December 1984, Mum, Dad and my sisters went on a camping trip to Woody Head, a picturesque seaside camping ground in northern New South Wales. They were joined by their friends Ron and Gay and their daughter Shay. A few days into the trip Shay fell ill with measles and was admitted to Lismore Base Hospital, where she spent three days recovering. Mum had been experiencing more bleeding and hadn't been feeling well, so decided to accompany Gay to the hospital so she could get checked out.

The blood test returned a result Mum couldn't initially comprehend. It revealed she was, in fact, pregnant.

Aside from mild shock, Mum's first reaction was excitement. It didn't last long. Because of the previous trauma to her womb and current level of bleeding, the doctor in charge took it upon himself to book a termination for the following day.

Back in those days, 36 was considered fairly old to have a baby, and the doctors simply didn't believe Mum could carry the pregnancy to full term without significant, if not fatal, complications.

'I was stunned,' Mum recalled. 'I asked if I could at least have an X-ray to determine the problem, but was told that Radiology wouldn't be available until Monday.'

Mum persuaded the doctors to cancel the termination until she'd had a chance to return to the campsite to discuss things with Dad. Mobile phones were still in their infancy, so driving back to Woody Head, nearly an hour away from the hospital, was the only option. They were reluctant to discharge Mum, and asked her to sign a document indemnifying the hospital against any and all consequences of not undergoing the termination, worried she might die on the way back home to Sydney.

'I thought about the children I'd brought into the world,' Mum explained, 'and knew I could never consider the possibility of not having them. Having Gay beside me strengthened my resolve, as she and Ron had adopted their two children after many long years of waiting, so the idea of terminating a pregnancy was abhorrent to them.'

Dad was also relieved when Mum got back to Woody Head and told him of the pregnancy. 'There was no way I would have agreed to a termination,' he recalled.

And eight months later, I arrived.

Mum said I looked almost identical to Eric when I was born. 'Dark skin, perfect features, tall and the same weight as your brother,' she often told me.

I'll be forever grateful to Mum for putting my own life before hers, and taking a risk despite being told the odds of my survival were slim.

Did I have the same, selfless resolve?

A Model Upbringing

It's ironic that I ended up reporting on fashion, as I started life with a passionate dislike for clothing. Until I started preschool, I was barely seen in anything bar a nappy and the occasional pair of sneakers. I did, however, have a penchant for plastic costume jewellery, which I would wear proudly as I made mud pies in the backyard of our family home and befriended the neighbourhood ducks. I was a nymph—a quiet little spirit with a deep connection to animals. One day when I was about five years old, I walked through the front door with a young magpie perched on my shoulder. 'Mum, this is my new friend, Melissa,' I proudly declared.

After nearly falling over, Mum suggested we go back outside, 'so Melissa can find its mum again'. *And not shit all over the house.* But the bird refused to leave my side for a week. I spent hours digging for worms to feed her, and made her a small makeshift house out of boxes on our second-floor balcony. The balcony was shaded by a group of tall gum trees, which Melissa could fly off to if she wanted to be with her bird family again. When a lady from WIRES, the local wildlife rescue service, came to take Melissa back to her family a few days later I cried and cried, feeling as if I'd lost my best friend.

I've always had an affinity for animals, and was born with an instinct to defend and protect the underdog, whether it be a friend who has been betrayed by their partner, or a pet dumped by their owner.

My childhood love of animals, bugs and dirt offered my parents a reprieve from the emotional dramas they were dealing with courtesy of my two pubescent sisters, Amy and Martine.

When not entertaining myself outdoors, I was in my cubby-house, reading. My parents encouraged me to read from a very early age, and I picked it up fairly quickly.

Mum often recalls the moment she realised I would likely have a future in words. I was three years old—and while I do take many of my mum's stories with a grain of salt, she swears I picked up a copy of my sister's *Vogue* magazine and started reading out loud. I could spend hours hibernating among blankets in the space beneath our home's staircase—which I had closed off with a beige, queen-sized bed sheet—getting lost in the worlds of Roald Dahl and Enid Blyton, imagining I was climbing the Faraway Tree with my friends Jo, Bessie and Fanny or living in a giant peach.

I was a very calm, independent child, and aloof, like my dad Ross. But I was also a worrier. When I was seven I spilled oil all over the terracotta tiles on our front terrace. The oil caused the porous tiles to stain, but the marks were only visible when it rained. I kept it a secret from my parents for almost a year, panicking to the point of tears every time the weather threatened a downpour, convinced I'd be disowned if Mum and Dad found out what I'd done. But when I finally built up the courage to tell Mum about my act of vandalism, she barely reacted. I'd spent a year of my life praying for sunshine, hiding what I thought was a terrible crime, only to have my indiscretion waved off with a 'Don't worry about it, darling.'

My anxiety was in its early stages, and followed me like a faint shadow through my adolescence, before eventually manifesting itself into a dark, electrically charged cloud which constantly threatened to break and shower me with panic.

Aside from my tendency to worry, I was a happy child. My childhood was idyllic, and I feel so blessed to have grown up in Newport, a safe, tight-knit community on Sydney's Northern Beaches in a modern, waterfront home the colour of pale pink fairy floss. We affectionately still refer to it as 'the pink house'. When summer rolled around we would spend weekends on Dad's boat, exploring the remote, tiny beaches punctuating the rugged coastline of Ku-ring-gai Chase National Park.

We also took a lot of road trips. When my sisters were young and I was a baby, my parents would take our caravan up the coast with a bunch of other families. I don't remember those trips, but from the photos—and Mum and Dad's stories— I knew I spent most of the time playing in mud or chasing unsuspecting native animals that had accidentally wandered into the caravan park. My bathtime consisted of a soap-free hose-down or a bath in the communal bathroom sinks before dinner, which was usually an outdoor affair lit by citronella candles. We'd dine on pork chops, charred sausages and potatoes baked in foil, while chatting and listening to the hum of cicadas as they were slowly replaced by a chorus of crickets, frogs and hungry fruit bats.

When I was about ten Dad traded in the caravan for a motor home and took Mum and me travelling around Australia for four months. We visited some amazing places: Katherine Gorge, Mataranka Springs, Uluru and Broome. Unfortunately my passion for reading—*Goosebumps* was my obsession at the time—caused some friction during the trip. On the 500 km drives between destinations I was the perfect child, too busy turning pages to ask 'are we there yet?'—but Dad was not impressed when I'd plead 'just one more chapter' as he pulled over to show us the latest waterfall, monument, memorial or giant ant nest he'd discovered at the latest stop on our bitumen adventure.

By the age of twelve, my tomboy tendencies had slowly, almost imperceptibly, faded, replaced by a love of glittery butterfly clips, bikinis and the Backstreet Boys. I idolised my older sisters, who were then in their early twenties. My parents had recently sold our Newport home and moved to a five-acre property in Ingleside. The small rural community, which neighboured Ku-ring-gai Chase National Park, was close to the Bahai Temple, a towering white dome-topped building which signalled drivers heading from the North Shore that they would soon arrive at the beachside suburb of Mona Vale.

The house itself was a 1970s five-bedroom, single-storey construction with a dark brown brick facade. A fireplace in the living room was our saving grace in winter, as the home's grey slate floor pulled the heat out of even the most Ugg-boot insulated feet, like a magnet.

Almost every block on the street was acreage, with twisting driveways so long that most homes couldn't be seen from the road. Signs offering free horse poo were dotted along the street, and horses would wander up to their enclosure fences hoping to score food from passers-by. Our house was sandwiched between paddocks and an Animal Welfare League shelter, which I ended up volunteering at in my mid-twenties.

As much as I liked the space the new home offered, I missed our pink house, with its soft, pastel carpet, glossy eucalyptus-hued cupboards and proximity to my school friends. We were only a few kilometres from Mona Vale's busy shopping centre, but taxis, buses and every single pizza shop on the Northern Beaches refused to come near our place. Being thirteen and unable to drive was torturous. I felt like I'd moved to Mars.

For Dad, who was a production engineer and inventor, our new digs could not have been more perfect. He suddenly had five acres to play with, and even before we moved in, he had built an enormous green shed on the front lawn. In fact, you could have easily run a large manufacturing business in it. It's the first thing that comes to mind when I picture my dad. During my childhood if I couldn't find him in the shed or the garage tinkering with a mate's car or fixing some kind of machinery, he would usually be in his study, looking through car magazines or the classifieds for more old, broken thingamajigs he could buy and fix.

His hands have always looked a decade older than the rest of him, and over the years have developed a distinct smell of car oil. One finger is shorter than it should be—the result of a run-in with a meat grinder—and every inch of skin bears some callus or scar.

I always look out for Dad's green shed when I'm flying out of Sydney, as it's so big you can easily spot it from the air. Dad's monster shed fit the campervan, a car hoist, a dozen shelving units filled with various tools and chemicals, two ride-on lawn-mowers, and still had space to spare for the flotsam and jetsam that inevitably returned with my sisters each time they broke up with a boyfriend or moved back home, occasionally with said boyfriend in tow.

It was Dad who first planted the idea of a career in journalism in my mind. One day, when I was about thirteen, he asked me what I'd like to be when I finished school. 'I'd like something to do with words, but I'm not exactly sure what that would be,' I said.

'Why don't you think about being a journalist, then?' Dad suggested. 'You could travel the world writing stories. When I was growing up, all the best movies I used to watch were about newspapers, because that's where all the action happened.' He rattled off films like *Superman*, *Citizen Kane* and *All The King's Men*. I'd heard of one of the three.

'Yeah, ok, cool,' I said non-committally.

◆ ◆ ◆

I loved having my sisters home, when they were in between boyfriends or affordable apartments. Being nearly a decade older than me, they were more like mothers than siblings, but I worshipped them and thought they were the coolest girls on earth. They'd let me raid their magazine stashes, and sometimes I'd borrow their clothes and organise photo shoots with my girlfriends using a cheap film camera I got in a show bag at The Royal Sydney Easter Show. My sister Amy was a successful model in her late teens and early 20s, travelling to Asia to shoot catalogues and ad campaigns. It seemed so glamorous and fun—being photographed in beautiful clothes, having your hair and makeup done and travelling to far-flung places.

So when, at the age of thirteen, at a fashion and lifestyle expo with my mum and sister, a model scout asked me to enter a modelling competition, I instantly said yes—even though I had no idea why she considered me. I was dressed in a black singlet and baggy khaki corduroy pants, my shoulder-length hair unwashed. Looking back, I realised she would have barely noticed my outfit—she simply saw a tall, skinny teen with clear skin. I didn't end up winning the Cleo Model Search, but it did lead to a contract with Vivien's Model Management.

Immediately after my first meeting with the agency, Mum took me to a Double Bay boutique to buy me a pair of high heels.

I'd practised walking in front of my new agent in a pair she had under her desk, and failed miserably. Rather than a runway star in the making, I resembled a newborn gazelle, wobbling around the desks trying my best to avoid face-planting against the wall of comp cards. 'We're going to need to work on her walk,' the agent murmured to my mum.

The new heels were black and glittery and cost about $300, an exorbitant sum. I'd never owned anything so expensive, or so pretty, and for weeks afterwards I spent hours admiring them in their box, almost too scared to practise walking in them and risk damaging their towering, spindly heels.

Mum was very hesitant about letting me model. She said I could as long as it didn't interfere with my schoolwork, and she came with me to every job and casting. If I reached a point where I didn't feel I was having fun, she told me, I had to stop.

I later learned that Amy had almost been kidnapped in Japan during a modelling trip when she was eighteen. She and another model had had their drinks spiked at a bar, and it was only due to the kindness and quick thinking of one of the bar staff, who snuck them out the back and put them in a taxi, that they made it back to their hotel before the date-rape drugs kicked in. They spent the next ten hours lying on the floor, unable to move. Mum booked a flight home for Amy as soon as she found out what happened, and told the Japanese agency to 'stuff their contract'.

I had a portfolio made up, and my own comp card. A comp card is an A5 sheet featuring your measurements and a selection of images you give to casting agents at go-sees. You show them your portfolio, then give them a comp card to keep, and cross your fingers you fit the bill.

My comp card said 'in development'. It was unlikely I would do much actual modelling for a few years, but agencies liked to sign up girls they thought had potential, almost like a lay-by so other agencies didn't scoop them up when they reached their mid-teens. I went to a few castings in school holidays, as my school was very strict on attendance, and was asked to visit my agency every few months, just to keep in touch. Looking back, I can see it was to make sure I wasn't becoming too curvy as I entered puberty.

About 18 months after I signed with Vivien's, Mum and I visited the agency again. The booker looked me up and down, eyes resting on my newly acquired hips and bust, and after a few pleasantries, told me I needed to lose weight.

'A few hours on the treadmill each week and some salads will do the trick,' she said.

Mum nearly punched her out.

I got home and devoured an entire pizza, and that was the end of my brief modelling career.

In any case, I don't think I would have coped well as a model. I always found it hard to deal with rejection, or to accept that I was simply 'not the right fit' for a job.

As well as being fiercely protective of her daughters, my mother was incredibly selfless. She spoiled us—our needs and desires before her own. I always had money for lunch orders and recess. Mum would pop a $2 coin in my hand as I got to the school gate. It was enough for a sausage roll and an orange and mango ice block, but occasionally I would have to buy one of the school bullies her own sausage roll, or risk being ousted from my group of friends.

I was spoiled, but I wasn't a brat. Shy? Yes. Aloof? Absolutely. But never disrespectful. I was always extremely grateful to Mum when she broke out the credit card, and never threw a tantrum if I was denied. As we grew up my sisters and I would chide her for it, blaming her and Dad for failing to properly prepare us for the realities of life. We grew up thinking we could have, and do, anything we wanted. The twenty-something comedown for each of us was cruel.

If you asked my dad, Mum's unwavering devotion to us led to the breakdown of their marriage. 'Don't neglect your husband when you have kids,' Dad said to me shortly after my wedding. 'Your mother practically ignored me when you were all born. I became the lowest priority and it ruined us.'

But the older I got, the better I understood Mum's reasons behind her desire to have us want for nothing.

She didn't want her daughters growing up feeling unloved and unwanted. She didn't want us to feel how she herself had felt as a child.

Neighbours

January, 2005

Nick was pissed off. It was warranted, I'm now happy to admit. It was summer in Bondi and finding a parking space anywhere near the beach was akin to winning the lottery. I had just moved into an apartment with my best friend Sarah, one street back from Sydney's famous Bondi Beach, and had managed to start a blue with my new neighbour before I had even unpacked my wardrobe.

He'd knocked on our door angrily, and the moment Sarah opened the door he growled, 'Did you park in my space again?'

'Sorry,' said Sarah. 'It's my new flatmate's car. She just had to bring some of her stuff in and we got distracted and forgot to move it.'

I was sitting in the lounge room listening to Sarah being grilled by this imposing, blue-eyed young man, trying not to bring attention to myself. Nick peered past Sarah and caught my eye.

'I'm so sorry, I had no idea it was your spot. It won't happen again,' I said, smiling gingerly.

Nick was suddenly a little disarmed. 'It's bloody hard to get parking around here, and I just got home from work, and it's really annoying when I can't park in my own car space,' he said, the edge in his voice dropping away.

'I know, I'm really sorry. Nice to meet you, anyway. My name's Elle.'

'Yep, hi,' he replied with a small smile, and shut the front door.

It wasn't an ideal start to my tenancy.

A week later I began tweaking our run-down, 1960s blond-brick apartment into something a bit more comfortable. I re-grouted the bathroom tiles, gave it a new coat of fresh white paint and attempted to rid the walls of the nicotine, scuff marks and grime we had inherited from dozens of previous tenants. I've always been my happiest when immersed in a project; something to work on, someone to fix.

I'd brought my white paint sample pot onto the balcony to paint our railing, which had once been white but was now mainly exposed metal with the odd flaking paint patch. Our landlord wasn't exactly proactive when it came to maintaining the apartment block, so if there was something broken or damaged, the only option was to fix it yourself or move out.

I heard Nick's balcony door open. He peered around the joint wall, and waved hello.

We spoke for a while, breaking the ice after the awkward car space incident. 'Would you mind painting your side of the railing?' I asked, handing him the small pot and wet paintbrush. He promised to do it when he got a spare moment.

I would never have guessed that just a few months later, I'd be painting it myself.

◆ ◆ ◆

It didn't take Nick and I long to move past our unpleasant introduction, and we soon became friends. I looked forward to hearing the whoosh of his balcony door open in the afternoons, as I sat on my unit's balcony ledge catching the last rays of the afternoon sun, the only time it hit our south-facing home.

If Sarah and I weren't having drinks with friends on a Saturday night, Nick and his flatmate Berg were, so we would head next door for a while before we went out.

I clearly remember the first time I realised my feelings for this tall, ash-haired neighbour were far from platonic. I was passing by the car park on my way to get a coffee one morning and spotted Nick talking to a tall, gorgeous blonde. As I waited for my cappuccino I realised I had suddenly fallen into a bad mood. It didn't take long to realise why: I was jealous! My jealousy soon turned into mortification, when Nick waved me over as I returned to the unit block.

'Hey Elle, this is Christina, my sister,' he said.

I was shocked by my feelings. I'd never really been in a serious relationship, and tended to fall for guys who were far from boyfriend material. My long-term idea had always been to stay single until my late twenties, as I had plans to wander the globe as a photographer and reporter for *National Geographic* magazine, and that lifestyle didn't lend itself to romantic commitment.

◆ ◆ ◆

Not long afterwards, Nick asked me on a date. He took me to Hurricane's bar and grill, just around the corner from our apartments. Over red wine and pork ribs, Nick told me more about himself. He grew up in Strathfield, and worked with his dad in the property industry. I've always felt you can tell a lot about a person from the company they keep, and Nick had the most solid group of great friends. They were all just really lovely guys, and would have done anything for each other.

Our relationship moved at record speed. We spent every day together, and were basically living together, a thick brick wall the only thing separating us. And within the space of just a few weeks, I was convinced Nick was The One. He was the guy I was going to marry.

This wasn't in my life plan, though. Not. At. All. I had too many adventures ahead of me, too much to achieve in my career to be worrying about relationships. I wasn't supposed to meet Nick until I was 27. *That* was when I wanted to start thinking about marriage, and babies, and all that stuff.

But I knew this guy was meant to be in my life—and if that was right now, then so be it.

◆ ◆ ◆

Nick and I could not be more different. I'm a cat person, he loves dogs. He's a big skier, I love a summer vacation. Nick's good at maths, but I prefer English. Nick loves carb-heavy Italian food,

I'm into Asian cuisines. Even our star signs are opposite: he's an Aquarian and I'm a fiery Leo.

Whenever Nick's mates are looking for something to do on a Saturday night, they know all they have to do is give him a call and he'll be up for a party. He just loves people. He's attentive, loyal to a fault, and has a charisma that makes it hard for people not to fall for his charms. I, on the other hand, love nothing more than curling up on a weekend with a book and a cup of tea, and find the company of animals much more comforting than people. I'm quite shy, and often feel awkward and anxious at social events. I think it's because I worry I'm going to get someone's name wrong, or say something stupid.

But for all our differences, over the years Nick and I have brought out the best in each other. Nick has become more intro-spective, and I, in turn, have become more confident socially. We constantly challenge each other to be our best selves, and I couldn't imagine my life without him.

I often think about that 'sliding doors' moment, when I decided to move to Bondi rather than follow Mum and my sisters to Brisbane. I had just spent a year living alone in Ultimo while I studied journalism at Macleay College, and was considering mov-ing up north to live with Mum while I figured out my next move.

Mum had moved to Queensland shortly after she and Dad had divorced; she couldn't bear to run into him, or their old friends, at the local supermarket. She had a new life, but was still constantly shadowed by her old one. Like a newly formed scab, a glimpse of Dad's car, or his new wife Suzette's car, was enough to scratch it off; make the emotions raw again.

Both of my sisters had moved to Brisbane. Amy and her husband Kristian were looking to escape the hedonistic rock-and-roll lifestyle they had lived for the best part of a decade, courtesy of Kristian's work as the drummer of well-known band, Grinspoon. Martine had split from her long-term boyfriend Gawain and wanted a fresh start, but he'd pursued her up north and they had moved back in together shortly after.

When I was accepted into Macleay College, I started looking for a city apartment. I knew myself too well to believe I'd commute to the city and back from Mona Vale every single day, and the college was strict on attendance: miss eight days or more and you're out. I found a modern one-bedroom apartment close to Sydney's Central Station. It was perfect, but too expensive.

'The cost is fine, honey,' Mum said to me after we left the inspection. 'I know you're going to do really well at Macleay, so I don't mind investing in your education by helping with the rent.' She gave me a long hug. 'I'd do anything for you, Elle. I am so proud of you.'

I didn't know how much Mum had received after her divorce settlement, but paying my rent for a whole year was a stretch. Still, she wouldn't take no for an answer. We had grown so close in the previous five years, just the two of us living together in Mona Vale, with our ginger cat, Cruikshanks.

I'd seen her at her lowest. I'd helped her bear the weight of the crushing depression which had settled inside her—seen my once lively, charismatic mother become a hollow shell, mimicking life without really living.

My parent's separation was a slow, painful process, like they were being sliced apart by a blunt knife, and something they initially tried hard to protect me from.

◆ ◆ ◆

A Mother's Choice

My six years in the cockroach-infested unit block above the old Bondi Fresh fruit shop were the most fun, exciting years of my life. When I moved in I was working as a promoter for Merivale's Tank nightclub. I'd spend my weeknights visiting bars around Sydney, handing out free entry and drink cards to people I'd meet and putting their names on the door for the coming weekend. I'd head into Tank at about 10 p.m. every Friday and spend the next six hours organising free drinks for regulars, chatting to guests and dancing to Martin Solveig and Eric Prydz tracks and the talents of DJs like Frankie Knuckles and Mousse T. About a year after quitting, I'd still get phone calls from drunk strangers at 1 a.m. asking me to put their names on the door.

Nick hated my job. We'd only just started dating and hadn't yet established a comfortable level of trust, so the idea of me having to befriend random guys, invite them to a bar and shower them with free drink passes irked him. He would come along to the nightclub and stand on the staircase for what seemed like hours, just watching me and waiting for 4 a.m., when I finished my shift.

I quit soon afterwards. A family friend of Nick's parents then offered me a job at Civic Video in Coogee. Each morning I'd put on my red Civic polo shirt and black pants, and get in my 1985 Honda Civic, which smelled so strongly of vomit it became a running joke among my friends. I had inherited the car from Amy, a few years after Dad bought it for a ridiculously cheap price. Dad loved an automotive bargain, and was great at sniffing one out, but unfortunately his nose didn't pick up the acrid stench that had settled itself into the upholstery courtesy of its previous owner, who must have let a bottle of rancid milk explode on the back seat. Clearly, his engineering mind had been distracted by its solid engine and reasonable mileage, but it was certainly the only feature Amy and I noticed. One day a friend of my sister's borrowed it for the day. It came back with a dozen Little Trees paper air fresheners hanging from the rear view mirror. It still didn't mask the rank mystery odour—it now smelled like someone had vomited in a pine forest.

I didn't love my job at Civic, but my plan to become a famous journalist was taking much longer than I had imagined. The unsolicited show reels and resumes I'd been sending to TV networks and magazines hadn't attracted any responses. But I was a hard worker, and the video store wasn't half as bad as my very first job, mopping floors and cleaning out the smelly display cases at the local fish and chip shop. At Civic, I'd actually look forward to Mondays, when a delivery of new-release DVDs arrived and I could prep them for rental. I'd open the boxes, remove the plastic from each DVD case, then place the *$5 a night rental* stickers and barcodes on each case with the care and precision of a master craftsperson before placing them on the shelves. It was a welcome distraction from the torturous 'See It At Civic' jingle that played on repeat on the TVs strung around the store. The song still haunts me, and I can still sing it verbatim.

It was during my time at the video store that I experienced the beginnings of full-blown anxiety. I had been invited to a job interview at Bare by Rebecca Davies, a high-end Sydney fashion label I loved. Being paid to steam silk dresses would be much better than stacking DVDs while I looked for my dream media job!

The interview was taking place an hour after I finished my shift. A few hours beforehand, I started to feel as though I was coming down with something. A nauseous feeling in my gut became so severe that I wondered if I was going to have to cancel the interview, which would have made such a poor first impression. *Suck it up Elle, just go and you can be sick afterwards,* I thought as I got into my car and headed for Paddington. As I was driving up Arden Street I felt like I was going to pass out. My heart began beating faster and faster, and my forehead and palms began to sweat. I pulled into a side street, got out of the car and almost fell into the gutter. I took my phone out of my handbag and called Nick.

'Something's wrong with me, Nick—I think I'm having a heart attack!' I sobbed. 'I've got an interview at Bare in half an hour and I don't want to tell them I can't make it—but I think I'm dying.'

'Take deep breaths,' he said. 'Just call them and tell them you have to go to the doctor right now, and I'm sure they'll be ok about it. You'll be fine, you're just panicking.' I called the manager, and she was very understanding and happy to reschedule. In the end, I went for the interview the following week and got the job.

Nick has always had a much cooler head than me. And he was right about the panic. I wasn't dying and I didn't have a heart problem, I discovered at the medical centre that afternoon. I'd just had a panic attack. Knowing what it was instantly calmed me down.

But having felt so helpless and out of control had been horrendously scary, and I prayed this would be my first and last experience with this horrible problem.

Little did I know it was just the start of my decade-long battle with anxiety.

A Million Splinters

Spring, 2002

My parents separated when I was fourteen. I was in year nine at the prestigious Pymble Ladies' College, a school that enforced super-strict rules about everything from the width of students' hair ribbons to the height of their socks. It had taken some time for me to settle in at the North Shore private school, having grown up thinking footwear was optional, and homework was something you did if you got home from the beach early enough.

Going through puberty was hard, but being stuck in the middle of my parents' messy divorce at the same time had a long-lasting effect on my mental health.

Two years after the split, Dad married my mum's best friend. Being the youngest and only child who couldn't move out and away from the drama, I became the collateral damage in this unfortunate love triangle.

On a clear, spring morning in 2002, the now fragile image I'd held of our slightly splintered family finally shattered into a million little pieces.

I woke up to the sound of silence. The usual, familiar noises of Mum's morning ritual—the cigarette-induced coughs and the tinkling metal spoon as she stirred sugary white tea in her delicate porcelain teacup—were absent. Mum rarely let me sleep in past 10 a.m. during school holidays, gently rapping on the door at about nine so I didn't sleep through an entire day, which I'd been known to do.

I roused myself, and padded down the beige-carpeted hallway of our small Mona Vale townhouse, and knocked on her door. Nothing.

After a pause, I opened it. She was in bed, lying so still.

'Morning, Mum,' I whispered.

Mum prided herself on her neat sleeping ability, boasting how easy it was to make her bed in the morning as every sheet was still neatly tucked in from the night before. But her sleep seemed different this morning. It was deeper, her chest inflation almost imperceptible beneath the thin, pale blue blanket. I walked over to her bed. 'Mum, wake up,' I said, louder.

Still no reaction. A sense of dread began to rise up from my toes. Something wasn't right. She'd been fine the night before.

A bit sad, but physically fine. We'd watched an hour of Fashion TV together and played a game of Scrabble, and I'd gone to bed just before her.

I shook her thin right shoulder, and felt her muscles contract ever so slightly. 'Mum!' I said loudly. She stirred, and tried to speak, but only managed a low moan.

'I'm calling Dad!' I said, breathlessly, racing downstairs and grabbing the cordless phone. I dialled Dad's mobile on the way back upstairs, but let it drop to my side as I reached the landing outside Mum's bedroom.

Mum was walking towards me, slowly. She was dressed in one of her thin, white cotton nightgowns, her eyes unfocused and bloodshot.

She was weaving between the hallway cupboards and the staircase railing, the sun beaming down from the overhead skylight giving her the appearance of a drunken angel. She was trying to talk, but every word was twisted and slurred, as though mangled through a washing machine before reaching my ears.

'Elle,' she managed, reaching her hand out towards me and stumbling towards the staircase. 'It's ok, honeh, I'm fi—.'

I heard the faint sounds of a man's voice coming from the cordless handset and put the phone back up to my ear.

'Mum's sick, hurry up and get here,' I said, and hung up the phone.

I took Mum's hand, walked her back to her room, and helped her back into bed, despite her muffled attempts at protest.

'Didn't take many . . . promise,' she whispered as she fought against her body's insistence that she sleep. 'I'll be fine, juss tired, don' call your father.'

A Mother's Choice

I waited in the hallway until Dad arrived. I couldn't look at Mum anymore. I didn't want to see her as vulnerable, this woman who had carried me through life up until this point. She was *my* rock; she wasn't supposed to crumble.

I was angry. I felt abandoned by my father, and all of the emotions I'd repressed over the past few months began bubbling to the surface as each minute passed.

I heard Dad open the front door and start up the stairs. I walked into Mum's room to let her know he was coming in.

She started to cry.

What happened next shocked each one of us in that small, shuttered room.

A growl escaped my lips and I launched myself at my father like a rabid animal. 'I hate you!' I screamed, throwing my fists towards his face. He grabbed my arms before I could make contact. My skinny limbs were no match for his 186 cm frame. 'I never want to speak to you again, get out of my life!' I yelled, before slamming the door and racing down the stairs. I ran out the front gate of our apartment complex and sat, perched on the high terracotta brick fence, sobbing.

I'd never talked back to my parents. I was a polite child who had never even raised her voice, save for the odd shout down the aisle of the local supermarket to ask Mum what kind of bread she wanted.

Part of me wanted to run back inside and protect Mum—to say I was sorry for not keeping the pain away, and that from now on I would. But I also felt betrayed by her, that I'd been dragged into this emotional saga between two people I loved dearly, and who I wanted, more than anything, to be in love with each other again.

Mum had taken twice the recommended dose of the sleeping pills her doctor had prescribed. She insisted she wasn't trying to kill herself, but I don't think at that point in time—when she was at her lowest—she would have minded if she never woke up.

◆ ◆ ◆

My relationship with Dad fell apart after that day. I knew enough about my parents' relationship to know he hadn't been happy for some time before their divorce, but also that the circumstances surrounding their eventual split had been handled badly by my father.

I would speak to him every few months, if that, for the next few years.

Not speaking to Dad crushed me. We had been so close, but he became almost a total stranger. One day, when I was at the local shopping village with my girlfriend Kristy, I saw Dad walking past, but didn't even acknowledge him. I was just so angry, and traumatised. I'd even distanced myself from his side of the family—my aunties and uncles and cousins; it upset me that Mum was no longer a part of their family functions. She and my sisters tried to encourage me to spend more time with them, but it would be years before I finally came back into their lives. It brought up too many emotions and memories of the times we all spent as one big, happy family, before everything became fractured. The Christmases we'd celebrated at Granny's house; searching the enormous artificial tree for sweets and little gifts bearing the names of my cousins and me; playing gin rummy using matchsticks to bet with, and drinking tea out of dainty porcelain cups like posh grown-ups.

One day in 2006 I received a call from Dad. We exchanged pleasantries, before, without any warning, he dropped a bombshell: he'd been diagnosed with prostate cancer.

I fell apart. My strong, stoic Dad, who I'd all but removed from my life, had cancer.

'I'm getting a radical prostatectomy, which will hopefully get rid of most of it,' he explained. 'I'll be getting it done at St Vincent's if you wanted to come and visit.'

I thought back to the time Mum had gone to Europe on a six-week vacation with my sisters, when I was still in high school. Mum arranged for me to stay with my best friend Prue and her family, explaining it would be easier to get me to school, while Dad stayed on his own at our home in Newport. I felt bad knowing Dad was on his own. *He'll be so lonely*, I thought. I cried almost every day that Mum was away, not because I was homesick, but because I worried about Dad being by himself for so long.

I felt that same worry as I took in the news of his diagnosis. I'd wasted four years—*we'd* wasted four years—barely speaking to each other, and I had no idea if we'd have another four years to make up for it.

Nick and I visited Dad at the hospital post-surgery. Nick had only met him a few times, and had been gently trying to coax me into spending more time with him.

It was the first time I'd seen Dad lying in a hospital bed. He looked so vulnerable, so old. I was so relieved when I heard that his prognosis was good, and that the surgeons thought they had removed all of the cancer.

For the first time in almost ten years, I told him I loved him. I felt my soul lighten as I kissed him on the forehead, and promised to call him when he was discharged from hospital.

It was the start of the reparation of our relationship.

Dad's never been much of a talker, like me, so it was much easier for both of us to sweep that part of our life from our minds and move on.

I recently asked him how he had felt during the years we lost touch. Had I asked Dad the same question ten years ago, he would have dismissed it, or twisted it into a conversation about Mum and all the reasons why their marriage was doomed. But whether it was illness, ageing or simply a broader perspective, Dad's response was surprisingly frank.

'I was devastated,' he admitted. 'I felt I let you all down.'

I saw his shoulders drop, and we both began to cry.

I hadn't realised I still harboured resentment until that moment, when I suddenly felt the acute absence of it.

That's Showbiz!

'Elle, you've bought *The Sun-Herald*,' laughed Nick when I got back from the supermarket. 'It's your competition!' I was so overwhelmed and excited that I hadn't been concentrating as I bought the Sunday paper I thought I'd soon be writing for.

'Shit, of course!' I said, looking down at the red masthead. I raced back downstairs and this time picked up the right paper, *The Sunday Telegraph*. A blue masthead. Blue for number one.

I couldn't believe that at the age of 21 I'd be working at the biggest-selling newspaper in the country. I would be taking coffee orders and sorting old newspapers, but it was a foot in the door and that was all I needed. I'd spent the past three years sending my resume and show reel to TV networks and magazines, trying to get a job—any job—in media.

I didn't care if I was writing about knitting needles or boat ramps, I just wanted to be part of a world that seemed so adventurous and exciting. And not having to slog it out at a regional or local newspaper covering school fetes and reporting on missing budgerigars was a huge bonus.

My recruitment had been unconventional, and very serendipitous. About a year prior, Christina had asked if I was keen to be interviewed for a story in *The Sunday Telegraph*. She worked in the public relations industry and a journalist she knew mentioned the paper was looking for case studies to illustrate a survey that had come out on Sydneysider's habits, and specifically wanted a young couple. At this time, I had started a job in marketing at a theatre production company in Balmain, which happened to be in the same building Nick worked in. (Nick at the time was working with his dad, who ran a property development company. I couldn't imagine Nick working in a more appropriate industry. He's a brilliant networker and negotiator, and has a very likeable, genuine demeanour like his dad.) Despite his misgivings, I roped Nick in to do the shoot with me. Nick is incredibly outgoing, but also very private.

'It'll take half an hour,' I told him. 'Please? No one will see it, it's a little story they're doing—and who knows, maybe I can persuade the guy interviewing me to give me a job.'

After a phone chat with Tony Vermeer, who was writing the story, Nick and I changed into our exercise gear and headed down the street to a nearby park to be shot by photographer

Dean Marzolla. The photo of Nick and I appeared on the front page of the paper that Sunday. It was the same week Australian model Michelle Leslie had been arrested in Bali on drugs charges, having been caught with ecstasy in her handbag. Our smiling faces appeared above a headline about her arrest.

At the time of the shoot I was three months into my theatre marketing career and hated it. I had a passionate dislike for musical theatre, and administration wasn't a strong point of mine. Several senior staff had also been quite intimidating, and after receiving more criticism than encouragement I had lost all confidence, ultimately causing me to make more and more mistakes. Two weeks before the *Sunday Tele* shoot my boss called me in for my probation review. She offered me another three months probation, but I'd had enough of dealing with grumpy old women and gave my notice.

Knowing my time in musical theatre was coming to an end, I brought my resume along to the shoot. 'I don't know if you can help, Dean, but are there any jobs going at the *Tele*?' I asked after the shoot. Dean promised to get my resume into the right hands.

Two days into my unemployment, Dean rang to say the editor was looking for a new copy kid, and would I be interested in applying.

I couldn't believe it. 'Of course!' I squealed. I had been so scared to leave my job with nothing to go to, but the universe had my back; I had just needed to take the leap into uncertainty, and free myself up for new opportunities.

I still remember what I wore to the interview: a black, knee-length pencil skirt and a pastel printed fitted jacket with slightly puffed shoulders.

Neil Breen, or 'Breenie' as the staff called him, conducted the interview, and while I can't remember a single answer to his questions, I left feeling hopeful and fairly confident. I had, up to that point, been given every job for which I'd attended a face-to-face interview, which I thought gave me pretty good odds.

A few days later I received a call back telling me I would be *The Sunday Telegraph*'s newest editorial assistant.

Pauline, who would be my immediate boss, was an older lady whose pastel twinsets and grandmotherly looks belied her steely disposition. I was warned in my first week that Pauline was much tougher than she appeared. She had a reputation for turning even the most senior reporter into a cowering mess if she caught them taking too many Post-It notes from the stationery cupboard. But I got along really well with Pauline. I did my job, and much more, and she in turn reserved her temper for other staff members.

On my first day I was introduced to Miawling, the former copy kid who had just been promoted to a cadet. She showed me the ropes, and took me through my responsibilities. My day-to-day tasks would involve fetching coffees and lunch for the editor and deputy editor on Saturdays, helping reporters with research, answering calls from readers, and delivering newspapers and mail each morning.

The best part of my job, however, was the chance to write. I was responsible for writing the Pet of The Week story, which appeared in the Funday children's lift-out, and writing the profiles for Babies and Weddings, which I was assured were among the most well-read sections of the paper. It was unlikely they'd get me nominated for a Walkley Award, but I would get a by-line, and it would be a good way to exercise my 'fluff' muscles.

I had always been more skilled at condensing information into small, bite-sized pieces than expanding and elaborating. I excelled at writing during high school, except when it came to essays. While other students would offer up fifteen pages of waffle, some simply hoping the marker would get too bored to read the entire thing and give them an automatic A for effort, I would hand in my two-page report on the underlying themes referenced in the course material, and the teacher would ask where the rest of it was. I always got marked down for my essay lengths, but was usually highly praised for their content. I resigned myself to the idea that perhaps photojournalism would be my calling in the media, rather than writing.

When I began studying at Macleay College, however, I discovered my short and sharp writing style wasn't a drawback. In fact, I aced my news-writing classes. 'You write very concisely,' my teacher told me one day, handing back a 300-word news story assignment. 'It's a great skill to have in newspaper reporting.'

Maybe I *would* consider print journalism after all, I thought. I did enjoy writing, and knowing my high school English shortcoming could be an advantage in the media gave me a newfound sense of confidence.

◆ ◆ ◆

I can't describe the pride I felt seeing my name in the *Sunday Tele* that first Sunday. I had taken Nick out to breakfast at our favourite cafe, flicked through to the middle of the paper and showed him my very first story—a profile on a tabby cat named Inca who was available for adoption at West Hoxton Animal Shelter.

'A shy but inquisitive kitty, Inca adapts well to new surroundings if given time to explore and he will become a friend for life once settled in,' the story read. It was the perfect yarn to launch my media career, considering my deep fondness for animals, particularly cats. If we weren't dating, I would have adopted Inca myself, except that Nick hated cats. But I felt sure my glowing summary would attract plenty of families who could give Inca a 'forever home'.

Another perk of my new job, I discovered, was the mail delivery. I couldn't believe how lucky some of the reporters were, especially the team who worked on the wellness lift-out Body + Soul. Some days their mail would fill an entire trolley, with giant boxes of hair product samples, super foods and peach- and strawberry-scented body washes.

Cushla Chauhan, Body + Soul's editor at the time, was one of the few reporters who gave me more than a sideways glance when I placed her papers on her desk each morning. She was so generous, and in exchange for hauling up the team's postal deliveries or writing small blurbs in the section, would leave bags brimming with products on my desk as thanks. As I became more senior at the *Telegraph* I adopted the same habit, often leaving product samples from events I attended at the editorial assistants' desk for them to share amongst themselves. I knew how unappreciated and invisible you could feel doing their job; many of them worked as hard, if not harder, than the full-time reporters, for a fraction of the salary.

It didn't take me long to notice the similarities between newspaper teams and the groups you would find at high school. You had the sports reporters, whose desks were decorated with Boonie dolls and football jerseys; there was a lot of backslapping and shouting when a major cricket or rugby match was on. There were the hyper-intelligent political reporters, who were very serious and tended to hoard old newspapers, piling them on top of one another like unstable Jenga towers. I'm still amazed none of them have become victims of a newsprint landslide. The sub-editing team could on occasion be quite grumpy—understandable considering they constantly dealt with sloppy grammar and stories that hadn't been proofread before they were filed.

It was easy to know you were passing the Insider lifestyle crew, as their area smelled like patchouli and jasmine, depending on which candle was burning at the time. The Insiders were much like the typical high school 'cool group'. They would whirr into the office after attending glamorous red carpet events or celebrity interviews, chatting loudly about who was hot and who was definitely not.

I decided within my first week at *The Sunday Telegraph* that I definitely wanted to be an Insider.

So I bought a corkboard and some glue sticks, took them home and got to work on a 'dream board'. I had always been a huge devotee of inspirational collages, having read way too many self-help books since my late teens. Tony Robbins, Wayne W. Dyer and Rhonda Byrne were my favourite motivational gurus. They all spruiked similar philosophies, throwing around phrases such as *If you can dream it, you can do it*, and *What you think about, you attract*.

I cut out the back page masthead of Insider, which at the time featured photos of Ros Reines, Melissa Hoyer and Richard Clune. I then cut out my own head from a happy snap I had recently taken, and stuck it up beside their professionally shot portraits.

'My photo is going to be up here one day, for real,' I said to Nick, showing him my handiwork. We both laughed.

I hung up my dream board beside my bed, so it was the first thing I saw when I woke up in the morning, and the last thing I saw when I went to bed. It also had pictures of wads of cash, and thin Victoria's Secret models jumping off a super yacht in the Mediterranean, but no matter how hard I wished, I never managed to grow three inches taller, ten kilos lighter and five years younger. But as the Rolling Stones sang, *You can't always get what you want.*

◆ ◆ ◆

I couldn't breathe. No, that wasn't it. I could complete the act of breathing, but it was the satisfying hit of oxygen, which is meant to occur with each inhalation, that just didn't come. I could breathe, but I couldn't *catch* my breath.

Every few intakes of air I would manage to overcome the feeling of asphyxiation; it was like a gate into my lungs finally crashed open, filling them with life-giving oxygen just in time.

I was 22 when, after years experiencing the odd panic attack, I developed full-blown anxiety.

I was at work, having celebrated my birthday just a few weeks beforehand, when it struck, seemingly out of the blue.

Nothing about my day had been extraordinary; there was no crisis or incident that triggered it. I was transcribing an interview I'd done that morning and noticed, as I sat at my desk and typed, a feeling of pressure on my lungs. It was light pressure, but enough to push my heart rate up. I tried to concentrate on my breathing, but rather than slowing my breath down, it made me even more aware of the trouble I was having getting air into my lungs. *This is not normal*, I thought. I stood up, then sat back down again, too lightheaded to stand.

This feeling was different to panic attacks I'd had in the past. I knew I wasn't dying, and the sweaty, frightened feeling I associated with panic attacks wasn't there. I just couldn't breathe properly.

And unlike my panic attacks, this didn't dissipate after an hour. In fact, it lasted a whole week. I couldn't function. I couldn't think about anything but my lungs, which seemed to have shrunk to the size of two small legumes, which, amazingly, were sustaining my life with just the bare minimum of oxygen filling their tiny capacities. It was frustrating, frightening and debilitating.

Convinced I had developed emphysema or asthma, I went to see Doc, asking for a lung test. The pulmonary function test was like a police breath test only much, much harder. The tube was the size of a bottle top, and trying to get enough force behind my breath for a confirmed reading was exhausting. After five tries my chest was on fire, but I managed one final exhalation and heard the beep of success.

'There's nothing wrong with them,' Doc said a little while later, after reviewing the results. It was all in my head.

The stress and worry I had been living with for years had all of a sudden become a physical manifestation—a chest-tightening, asphyxiating ball of anxiousness blocking my lungs.

Beta-blockers would be the best option from a medication perspective, Doc explained, but the best treatment couldn't be chased down with a glass of water. I needed to sort my mind out, he said, and suggested I consider seeing a counsellor.

After returning from what I dubbed a 'mental health week', and fearing I'd ruined my chances of career advancement, I arranged a meeting with Breenie. Who'd want to deal with an employee with a mental health problem? I imagined the word LIABILITY tattooed on my forehead, like a big neon sign warning Breenie I was unstable, as I walked into his glass office. My eyes glanced out to the open plan area, looking for signs people were watching our exchange; they would no doubt be wondering where I'd been for the past week. *Is she quitting? Is she going to be fired? Has she got some terminal illness?* I imagined my colleagues asking each other in whispered voices as I broke down in front of the editor.

I'll be forever grateful to Breenie for his understanding during that time. I was barely a blip on the staff radar, but he made me feel like an important part of the team. He recommended I see the company's counsellor. The sessions would be completely confidential, he explained, and I could take them any time I needed.

◆ ◆ ◆

'What's the worst that could happen?'

This question, posed by the counsellor, was a turning point for me.

I had explained that I often worried how I'd be perceived if I wasn't one of the first in the office each morning—that I'd be considered lazy, or not determined enough to make it as a journalist.

'If you got to work ten minutes late, which as you said is pretty unlikely, what's the worst that could happen?'

'I'd be told not to let it happen again?' I replied, unsurely. 'Or they'd fire me?'

'How likely is it that you'd be fired for turning up a bit late if your bus was delayed, and you were rarely at work later than 8.30 most mornings?' he asked.

'Pretty unlikely,' I conceded with a laugh.

The counsellor asked me to apply this question to other concerns I had about work and life, which would help put them into perspective. We practised some meditation and breathing exercises, and I left the session feeling a little lighter. My lungs had expanded slightly, the chest pressure easing and allowing me the satisfaction of a few full breaths.

I would continue to battle my anxious breathlessness for the next decade, but having an arsenal of tools made this beast much easier to subdue.

◆ ◆ ◆

On weekends before I landed my job at the paper, I would catch the bus to Bondi Junction and spend hours—sometimes the entire day—in the comfy armchairs of Borders bookstore reading titles on how to get that dream job. I loved reading career books as much as I enjoyed crafting together dream boards.

My bookshelf at home was filled with tomes such as *Nice Girls Don't Get The Corner Office, What Colour is Your Parachute?* and *Network Your Way to Success*. I would highlight quotes, scribble thoughts in my notebook and refine my resume using the tips offered up.

One piece of advice I came across during my Borders sessions was to dress for the job I wanted, not the one I had. If I dressed for the job I had, I should have worn comfy sneakers, jeans, and a dark-coloured top to hide the ink stains incurred from hauling piles of newspapers around the newsroom.

And so I dressed like a fashion writer. Designer threads were out of the question, on my meagre salary, but I did my best to dress the part, scouring vintage stores and markets on weekends looking for chic dresses and blazers. My go-to ensemble generally consisted of a knee-length, 70s-style rayon or polyester dress in a bold print complete with pussy bow, knife pleats or statement sleeves, over black stockings and a blazer or jacket. I would tie my shoulder-length hair up into a topknot or low ponytail and finish with a bright lip shade. (Looking at my wardrobe today, with its distinct lack of colour and print, you'd be excused for thinking you had gone colour blind!)

I cringe thinking back to some of the outfits I wore, but at the time I felt I was the epitome of chic and would soon be discussing the season's latest runway trends with Kirstie Clements, who was then the editor of *Vogue Australia*.

Fortunately magazines, which were definitely not an expense I could afford, could be found splashed over the desks of my more senior colleagues, and most of them were generous enough to hand them over once they'd flicked through. Melissa Hoyer, Ros Reines and the Insider editor Michelle Lollo would routinely offer me their copies of fashion magazines, which I would devour on the train home looking for inspiration for my wardrobe.

About two months into my tenure, I politely asked Pauline if I could sit in on the editorial team's weekly conference— provided, of course, that I'd done all my deliveries and jobs that morning. Each Tuesday the paper's reporters would pitch the stories they were working on to the editor and discuss ideas for that Sunday's edition. She reluctantly agreed.

It was great to get a feel for how the paper was put together, and what made a compelling new story. Breenie was an editor who knew what he wanted, and I came to realise there was a real art to selling a story in conference.

One day I approached my chief of staff, Miranda Wood, with a story idea. Part of my job was to open mail from readers and take calls from people with tips or feedback. One particular letter was from a lady complaining that there were very few stores where older women could find modern, fashionable clothing that didn't make them look like mutton dressed as lamb.

I mentioned this to my mum in passing during a phone call a few nights later, and she agreed with the letter writer. I sensed the beginnings of a story, did some research into the fashion offerings for baby boomers and decided to pitch my first story in conference.

When the Tuesday rolled around, I walked into the conference room with my shorthand notepad, and patiently waited until all the reporters had pitched their stories. Breenie seemed in a good mood, so I asked if I could offer up an idea.

'Female baby boomers are angry about the lack of fashionable clothing available to them,' I said, way too quickly. I had been rehearsing my pitch for two days, but still felt extremely nervous. 'They're the most cashed-up generation and have money to burn, but there are hardly any designers creating clothing to suit their post-menopausal body shapes, and they want this to change.'

A few minutes after the editors came out of their post-conference meeting, my chief of staff, Miranda Wood, approached my desk.

'Breenie loves the story,' she said. 'He wants to run it as a double-page spread, so we'll need about 700 words by Thursday.'

I blanched. At college we were given weeks to write stories that long. I would need to interview designers, a number of older women, and organise photo shoots for the piece. I worked until about 10 p.m. that night and the following day, trying to make the story worthy of two whole pages.

I was so thrilled when I opened *The Sunday Telegraph* that weekend and saw the story and my by-line. From that moment I knew I wanted to write about fashion and style—not just about pretty dresses and what was trending, but real news yarns that could make an impact on the industry.

After that, I wasn't just an observer at conference. I was encouraged, and then expected, to offer story ideas each week, and within a month was writing two to three stories per week on top of my editorial assistant duties.

I would arrive at the office by 7.30 a.m., so I could get a head start on my tasks, and had time to write and look for story ideas before having to fetch old papers from the library for lazy senior reporters or get them coffee. While most reporters knew not to ask certain things of the copy kids, lest they incited the wrath of Pauline, a few were brave enough to task us with jobs definitely not in our job description, such as opening their mail and topping up parking meters. Still, I went above and beyond when it came to my role. We were expected to fetch breakfast and coffee for the senior staff on Saturdays, the busiest day; I wanted the deputy and assistant editors to know me, so as soon as they arrived I would take their coffee and toast orders and ensure they started their day content and caffeinated.

In conference I became known for my quirky pitches. I didn't just write fashion pieces, but my ideas often punctuated the more serious crime and political stories with a splash of colour and fun. I brought a 'show-and-tell' element, bringing in photos of strange fashion trends that could make for an eye-catching picture story.

Tuesday conference wasn't all roses and group hugs, however. In fact, more often it was quite the opposite, depending on Breenie's mood. If the previous week's paper had a fabulous front-page splash or great exclusives there'd be plenty of laughs; if not, we would all know about it fairly quickly. If your story ideas were crap, he'd be sure to pull you up on it, usually in front of the entire editorial team. There were no grey areas with Breenie. You could walk out of conference feeling like the king of the world one week, and like a pariah the next. It was extremely tough on the nerves, but I appreciated the fact you always knew where you stood with him.

On top of my contributions to the general news section, I hounded the Insider team for jobs, hoping to land a by-line in the showbiz section. Occasionally I'd be lucky enough to snag an invitation to an event to cover for the social pages. Pauline didn't approve of her charges being given work by the section editors, unless it had been run past her first, but I really loved contributing to the party pages, so I'd sneakily attend events after work, write the copy before Pauline arrived the next morning, and cross my fingers she wouldn't notice my by-line beneath that Sunday's party write-up.

◆ ◆ ◆

Six months into my gig as an editorial assistant, I was offered a one-year cadetship. I couldn't believe my luck. I would no longer have to field angry telephone calls every time the price of the paper increased, or a newsagent hadn't been sent enough promotional bucket hats or miniature recipe book collections for the paper's readers.

At about the same time, Kate Waterhouse had been appointed *The Sunday Telegraph*'s Style writer. She had inherited the coveted column from Melissa Hoyer, who for years had filled the pages with sartorial snippets and juicy industry gossip.

Kate's profile was on the rise at the time. The daughter of racing identity Gai Waterhouse, Kate's polished style, friendly nature and socialite status saw her top the invite lists to every A-list party, and she was front and centre at every major racing event, as well as being David Jones' race-wear ambassador. Kate had been guest editing the paper's party pages for some time, and Breenie, who knew Kate well through his love of horseracing, decided to appoint her the new Style columnist.

Under Kate's direction, Style became more visual, offering trend-based pictorial spreads supplemented by fashion sales listings and fashion news.

In February 2009, almost a year into Kate's tenure, I was called into the office of the paper's then deputy editor, Helen McCabe. Helen's news sense was as impeccable as her blonde, shoulder-length blow waves, and she instilled in me equal amounts of awe and terror.

'How do you feel about pulling together the fashion pages from next week?' she asked me, skipping the small talk.

For a moment I was speechless. 'What? Um, I'd, I'd . . . *love* to!' I stammered.

'It would just be for a few weeks, until we find a permanent replacement for Kate,' she said brusquely, before ushering me out of her office.

I was never privy to all the details surrounding Kate's sudden departure, but I do know it wasn't due to her performance. And while I may have landed the job by default, if only for a few weeks, it was an opportunity I was thrilled with, and one I was damned determined to make the most of.

On my way home that day I stopped by a liquor store and bought a bottle of Veuve Clicquot. I felt like I had won the lottery, even though my temporary promotion hadn't included an increase in my very modest salary. My extravagant purchase significantly dented my weekly pay, but getting creative with pantry staples for a couple of dinners would be worth the splurge.

'How was your day?' Nick asked casually when he came home. He looked at the coffee table, which had been set up with the bottle of Clicquot, two champagne glasses and a decadent platter of French cheeses, quince paste, water crackers and his favourite Jatz biscuits.

'Not bad,' I said, trying to sound casual.

'Not bad considering I'm the new FASHION WRITER FOR THE SUNDAY TELEGRAPH!' I shouted, running up to him and throwing my arms around his neck.

'No way! That's amazing, Happy! Congratulations!'

Happy was Nick's nickname for me. He always said it was my happy disposition that he'd fallen for when we first met. He thought I was pretty, too, but there were heaps of hot girls in Bondi. 'But you're the hottest, *and* the happiest,' he'd tell me.

Later that night, after talking through my new job, I walked into our bedroom and sat on our creaky bed. I stared at my inspiration board, looking at the pasted Insider masthead that bore my makeshift photo. It had already begun to yellow.

I offered my glass up to the universe, and took a swig of its contents, letting its bubbly contents fizz amongst the butterflies that had set up residence in my gut.

My first column would be published a couple of weeks before Valentine's Day, so I decided to make that the theme of my main spread. I featured four runway images, each photoshopped over a backdrop of pink cherry blossom trees in bloom. I had absolutely no idea what I was doing, and I cringe now even thinking about it, but at the time I was so proud of myself.

I brought my debut fashion spread into Breenie's office and held my breath as he briefly scanned the two pages. 'It's very pink,' he quipped. If I wasn't still in a state of semi shock at my incredible new job, I would have noticed his lack of enthusiasm for my rose-hued column much more keenly. There were very few topics Breenie didn't have a complete grasp on, but fortunately for me, fashion was one of them. My column ran, and I bought about six copies of the paper that Sunday.

My appointment opened up a new universe. I'd gone from begging fashion and celebrity publicists to call me back about story ideas I had, to being chased by them. My desk started to pile up with invitations to movie screenings, fashion launches and beauty events, and I had designers wanting me to write stories about them.

Breenie and Helen hadn't given me the job because I was a last resort. I had proven I could sniff out good news stories and find interesting angles hiding in piles of press releases. They could have easily slipped in a fashion stylist while looking for an experienced replacement, but I think they hoped I might approach the section in a fresh, news-focused way. As a cadet, I'd sift through every section of the paper looking for interesting story ideas other reporters may have missed. Being completely unknown in the media and having zero contacts had forced me to be resourceful, and I'd become adept at finding yarns in the most unlikely places.

Once, while looking through the 'wanted' classifieds during my editorial assistant days, I found a listing someone had placed looking for the little stickers you find on fruit at the supermarket. I called the man who placed the ad, and discovered he had amassed Australia's most comprehensive collection of fruit stickers. I pitched it in conference, Breenie loved the quirky story and it ran that weekend.

My first few days as Style columnist were a whirlwind, and extremely exciting—but before I had even basked in the glory of my first published fashion spread, my confidence was squashed like an ant beneath a patent Jimmy Choo stiletto.

The Wednesday before my first column ran, a well-known fashion blogger had published a nasty story about 'The Sunday Telegraph's new Style writer'. She had never met me, and yet she felt it necessary to pen a cruel, sarcastic and belittling story about me. She'd dug up a piece on dogs I'd been asked to write as a cadet, in order to show I was unfit to edit the pages. I was devastated, certain everyone in the fashion industry was going to read it and think I was a dunce.

Sure, I was green, but who wouldn't have grabbed one of the most sought-after jobs in Australian media if it was offered to them? What I lacked in experience I made up for in effort and determination, and I was a quick learner and a competent writer.

Nick had never seen me so upset when I walked through the door that night, mascara running all over my face like a road map. 'I can't do it!' I wailed, putting my head in my hands. I wanted to run across the road, plunge headfirst into the Bondi surf and disappear.

'Elle, you're new to this,' Nick said gently after I'd stopped crying and explained what had happened. 'People are going to be jealous, and there will probably be plenty more who will try and make you feel unworthy, but you'll prove them wrong. You've just got to stick it out and keep working hard. Breenie and Helen wouldn't have given you the job if they didn't think you could handle it.'

I still occasionally cross paths with this blogger, and have been tempted to thank her. Her story added the first layer of armour that would eventually harden my once soft, sensitive disposition into something more suited to the dog-eat-dog world of print media.

◆ ◆ ◆

About a year into my appointment as fashion writer, I took a vacation to Bali. I'd taken just one holiday since starting at the paper, and my anxiousness was becoming worse and worse. I hadn't exercised in months, and was surviving on macchiatos and hot chips from the News Limited canteen.

A few days before I was due back at work, J.Mo gave me a call.

J.Mo at the time was the paper's newly appointed music writer. He had previously worked as an entertainment reporter for AAP, and before that had covered everything from crime to politics. During my first few months at the paper, I tried as hard as I could to avoid him. I found his loud personality and twisted sense of humour very intimidating, and quickly convinced myself he disliked me. I soon came to realise that, as odd as it sounds, J.Mo was actually more offensive to people he was fond of. If J.Mo was ever super-polite to someone, you knew there was a fight brewing.

'I think we're going to be working on something new together, babe,' J.Mo explained. 'I don't know too much about it, but Breenie's making some big changes to Insider, so don't be surprised if you get called into his office when you get back.'

Two days later I walked into work, and was ousted from the fashion column.

Mrs Harry Styles

I was livid. I'd worked my butt off on those pages, and had scooped a number of big fashion stories in the previous few months. I'd started to gain momentum and had been planning to pitch an idea for a new layout.

I held back tears as Breenie explained he wanted me to cover gossip with J.Mo under the new-look Insider section, which would launch in a few weeks.

Ros Reines had been covering that round for the paper for years and had developed a solid following. I knew people who bought the paper just to find out whose Sundays she had ruined.

Ros would now be writing an opinion-based column focusing on the salacious stories of Sydney's social scene, Breenie explained, but J.Mo and I would tackle the gossip round from an entertainment angle, writing about the antics of pop stars, actors and models.

I didn't want to do it, and was tempted to quit. I'd been at *The Sunday Telegraph* for almost three years, which for a Gen Y-er was a pretty long time. But there were still so many things I loved about my job—my colleagues, the opportunities to travel, and the excitement of the newsroom—so I let the feeling pass.

'The editor just asked me why the fashion writer gave him a death stare in the foyer,' my boss Kerry Parnell quipped when I returned from my lunch break later that day. I was flitting between sadness and fury, still unsure how to feel about this new role and the loss of my old one.

'Let me give you some advice,' she told me, lowering her voice. Kerry had edited several esteemed fashion magazines prior to being appointed the editor of Insider, and never lost her cool. 'Don't get emotional at work. If you want to get ahead, keep your feelings in check.'

And so I subconsciously added another steel layer to my growing armour, wiped my eyes and got on with writing what would be one of my final Style columns.

◆ ◆ ◆

Working with J.Mo was as intense as it was fun. He knew almost every publicist, soap star and pop singer in Sydney and had the little black book to prove it. An *actual* little, black, book. Despite my advice to enter the 21st century and store his phone numbers electronically, the A5 address book still sits, bulging at his desk, today.

He was permanently surrounded by famous people. He'd drag me to every party, making my head spin as he introduced me to dozens of industry insiders who he called 'Babes' or 'Darling'. It wasn't uncommon for him to drop me to my car after work with Casey Donovan—who was his flatmate at one point—or a *Home and Away* star sitting in the front seat.

Our personalities could not be more different, and his extroverted, emotional personality often clashed with my more reserved demeanor. I fought with him more than anybody I'd ever met—even my own family—but we cared for each other and shared more than a few adventures during our time on the 'J.Mo and Elle' column.

One of my more memorable 'J.Mo and Elle' moments happened during the very first Australian season of *The Voice*. The finals were in full swing, and J.Mo and I had been invited for a 'mani pedi' with *Voice* coach Seal and his final charges Karise Eden and Fatai at his hotel room.

We were allocated an hour with the US singer for our nail treatments, an interview and a photo. It didn't take long for us to realise that Seal—who is a very lovely guy—loves a chat. And I mean *loves* a chat. When he first began to talk about his final contestants and the advice he'd been offering them, I turned to glance at the two girls, and was appalled to see they were completely ignoring him. *He had decades of experience in the music industry, and so much to offer these novices*, I thought. Luckily, Seal didn't seem to notice their disinterest. In fact, I don't think he would have cared if *everyone* was ignoring him— he just kept on talking. About half an hour into his monologue, which had now morphed into a one-way discussion about the benefits of fasting, I started to see why his young mentees had tuned out. Our allocated hour had passed, and Seal was still talking. By this time we'd asked him all of two questions, and the News Corp photographer, Sam, began waving at us and gesturing to his watch, desperate to get his photo so he could rush to his next job. The show's publicity team were equally anxious to wrap up the pamper session, but it was virtually impossible to get a word in. At this point I actually felt sorry for Karise and Fatai, as this was definitely not their first two-hour chat session with Seal. After that meeting, every time a contestant on *The Voice* chose Seal to coach them, I couldn't help smiling just a bit, hoping they knew what they were in for.

◆ ◆ ◆

In 2012, a special issue of *Girlfriend* magazine dropped onto my desk. 'One Direction's in town and we're looking for an upfront entertainment story,' said Woodsy, my chief of staff at the time. 'J.Mo's away, so can you head down to Fox Studios and see if you can get a good news line from them?'

Despite my ousting from Style, I still mainly wrote fashion news stories for the paper. I'd built solid relationships in the industry, so many of the stories I pitched and wrote about in 'J.Mo and Elle' involved models, designers or fashion trends. J.Mo mainly covered the music and television side of things, but we would cover each other's rounds when one of us was away.

I'd heard about the British boy band, who had been sending Australia's tweens into an absolute meltdown since arriving in Sydney earlier that week. They had burst onto the pop scene

18 months prior, having placed third on the *The X Factor* UK, and their debut album *Up All Night* had shot to the top of the ARIA albums chart.

The teenage pop stars were performing to an intimate crowd of radio station prize-winners, and *The Daily Telegraph* had been offered an interview with them after the show.

With so many reality singing shows around these days, it's hard to stay on top of what the alumni from the Australian shows are up to, let alone the British and American versions, so my 1D knowledge was very minimal and I'd had no time to prepare. If Niall Horan had smacked me across the face on my way to the interview I would've had no idea who he was.

The interview was going to be filmed for the paper's website, so I sat studying *Girlfriend*'s One Direction Aussie Tour Special Edition outside the concert hall a few minutes before they began their performance, trying to remember my Louises from my Liams. I had very low expectations they would deliver much in the way of a page-three story. We'd received a tip that the boys had a habit of stealing items from hotel rooms, and this was probably my best bet, I thought, at getting an exclusive angle.

Luckily I'd arrived at work that day looking half decent. I had an appointment with a wedding dress designer that night with some girlfriends, so I'd straightened my shoulder-length blonde hair and donned a black, galaxy-print Josh Goot mini dress with black hosiery and a pair of towering black heels.

The boys were lovely and fairly polite, except Liam. He kept barking like a dog after Louis admitted he had a habit of 'borrowing' animal souvenirs from hotels they had stayed in. 'I borrowed it and then got caught borrowing it and we had to give it back because they called up management and cried about it,' Louis admitted. It was mildly funny, but far from a cracking story, and our baby-boomer readers wouldn't have given two hoots about it.

Straight after the lacklustre interview, I phoned Woodsy. 'Sorry, I don't have a page three for you,' I said apologetically, hoping the news desk could make changes to their newspaper layout.

A moment later, the band's publicist called me.

'This is really awkward, Elle,' she began hesitantly. 'But, erm, Harry wanted to know if he could have your number.'

Harry, one of the boys I just interviewed? One of the *teenage* boys I just interviewed? If it wasn't for the hesitation in her voice, I would have thought she was pranking me.

'Ah, no,' I said, a little shocked. 'I'm engaged and on my way to try on wedding dresses. But I'm very flattered.'

I hung up the phone, and immediately thought about calling the publicist back. Going out with Harry Styles would land me a front-page story, for sure. It would also bring the wrath of a few hundred thousand teenage girls, but I'd copped my fair share of online abuse and wasn't fazed about a few 1D death threats. But I knew Nick would be far from impressed if I gave out my phone number simply for the sake of a by-line.

Instead I called Woodsy back. 'Ignore my last phone call,' I said, waving down a taxi outside Sydney's Fox Studios and making my way back to the office. 'I think I might have something . . .'

I TURNED DOWN HARRY STYLES, the page-three story read, below a photo of me posing on stage with the five young pop stars:

I don't know whether Harry had noticed the diamond ring on my finger and chosen to ignore it or whether—and this is more likely—he's an 18-year-old boy who's not highly attuned to things like that. Anyway, even if I were interested in a date with the latest pop sensation, my evening was already fixed with a strictly unchangeable appointment—to try on wedding gowns.

The story was picked up by media agencies around the world, and the video of my interview with the group viewed on YouTube more than half a million times.

♦ ♦ ♦

A few months prior to my encounter with Mr Styles, Nick had asked me to marry him. We'd been dating for seven years, and for the past two I'd been eagerly anticipating the knee bend. He was certainly taking his time, despite perfect and romantic opportunities to do so. I was only in my mid twenties, but we'd already seen so many of our friends meet, get married and have kids, so I'd started to think maybe he just wasn't ever going to.

On Christmas Eve in 2011, Nick had suggested we go for brunch at popular Bondi Beach breakfast cafe, Trio.

'Sure,' I said, throwing on a T-shirt and a pair of tights.

'Can you wear something a bit nicer?' he asked. 'It's Christmas Eve!'

'Ugh, fine,' I muttered. I slipped into a lemon-hued summer dress and a pair of sandals, and tied my hair in a ponytail. Nick always loved it when I wore my hair up in a pony.

We watched Bondi Beach fill up with sunbathers and tourists as the summer day grew warmer, and enjoyed the cafe's specialty breakfast dish of truffle-scrambled eggs with prosciutto. Enjoying the people watching and the perfect weather, I failed to register how lucky we were to have scored a table at one of Bondi's busiest eating spots, on one of its busiest days of the year. Nick had secretly made a reservation a few days prior, but I was completely oblivious.

'I've heard there were whales off South Bondi this morning,' Nick said casually as we finished our breakfast. 'Let's walk around and see if we can see any.'

I pointed to my lack of appropriate footwear, but Nick was determined. 'Ok,' he said, 'how about this? We'll just walk to Mackenzies Point and then we can come back.' I begrudgingly agreed.

We wandered past the Bondi Baths and around the first small cove, known as 'The Boot'. Nick suggested we sit on the rocks for a while and watch the surf, so we sat down on a rock ledge a few metres from the footpath. It was then that I noticed Nick was behaving rather oddly. After a few moments I saw him reach into the pocket of his white shorts.

My heart jolted. *Oh my god, this is it!*

Time slowed down, but my brain sped up. *Maybe he's just pulling a tissue out,* I reasoned, feeling a pang of disappointment. It then occurred to me that December is not whale-watching season, so there was no way we were here to spot sea creatures.

My mind was racing so madly that I didn't even register that Nick was now facing me on bended knee.

'Elle,' he asked, 'will you marry me?'

'Of course, *yes!*' I gushed.

He presented me with a stunning emerald-cut diamond, flanked by two smaller rectangular stones, on a simple gold band. It couldn't have been more perfect.

We sat on the rocks for almost an hour, calling our families and debriefing about the lead-up to the proposal. 'Remember a couple of weeks ago when we went to your dad and Suzette's house for dinner?' Nick asked. 'I went up to the shed with your dad to ask for your hand—but as soon as I'd worked up the courage to ask him, he cocked his shotgun and asked if I wanted to help him shoot the feral rabbits on the front lawn. I didn't think it was a good idea to ask while he had a loaded weapon in his hands, so I called him up a few days later.'

I laughed so hard fresh tears sprung from my eyes.

Just less than a year later, on that same rabbit hole-pocked lawn, we wed in front of 170 of our friends and very large families. It was the most chilled day, thanks to my aunty Melissa who was our celebrant, our wedding planner and caterer Hayley, and the fact that neither of us cared less about the colour of the flowers or what the cake looked like.

I didn't blow the budget on my dress, choosing an off-the-rack strapless gown with a tulle skirt and a corset bust adorned with white feathers. It was nothing like the slim-fitting, modern dress I'd envisioned when I first began searching, but it was classic, fitted my pear-shaped frame impeccably and flattered my figure.

The day before the Big Day I'd also rushed into Bianca Spender and purchased a simple, Grecian-style white cocktail dress for the reception, which was a little easier to hit the dance floor in.

The ceremony was held in the back garden, and we had a marquee set up on Dad's tennis court, which featured a dozen long tables. Each was simply adorned with small jars of white flowers and hessian table runners, and at dinner became laden with sumptuous share plates of fresh pasta, salads and perfectly cooked salmon and beef. The wine was flowing, the food was good, we had great company and lots of fun music, and that's all that mattered to us. A friend of Nick's gave us brilliant advice in the lead-up to the Big Day: 'Make sure that at least every hour you both go outside and spend five minutes with each other, just being present in the moment and taking it all in.' It made us really slow down and appreciate how incredible the day had been.

We'd throw the exact same wedding all over again.

◆ ◆ ◆

If Robert Pattinson had asked for my number, instead of Harry Styles, I would've had a much harder time resisting. He's been my celebrity crush since he first shot to fame as Bella Swan's love interest in *Twilight*. At the office it was easy to find my desk, thanks to the life-sized cardboard cut-out of Robert's character, Edward Cullen, which I'd placed beside it.

In 2010, ahead of the release of *The Twilight Saga: Eclipse*, our newspaper was offered an interview with 'R-Patz' and my name was put forward for it straight away. I don't think anybody else would have dared put their hand up for it, lest they cop my wrath.

I've never really been star-struck during an interview with a celebrity. I admire a lot of them, but it doesn't take long to realise they're just ordinary people with extraordinary jobs. But I was frozen with nerves when I heard R-Patz say 'hello' after the publicist put me through to his number.

'H-h-hi is that Robert?' I stammered.

'Yes, it's me,' the soft, British voice replied.

I decided to get the creepy fan grilling out of the way first. 'Have you ever done an interview with a journalist who was a crazed *Twilight* fan? Not that I am or anything,' I lied.

'I think I've had one,' he mused. 'She was from Vietnam and she was having a full-on panic attack in the interview, which was quite funny.'

So far I'd managed to keep my cool—sort of—and at least I now knew I wasn't the only interviewer who'd been close to losing her shit about talking to a Hollywood demigod. And surprisingly, he was one of the most lovely interviewees. I even helped him track down an old school friend, Charlie, who had lost contact after moving to Australia. 'Tell him to call my mum,' Robert said, 'because he's probably still got that number.' I included his call-out to Charlie in my feature article, and sure enough, Charlie got in touch with Robert's mum a few days later.

I met Robert a year later at the premiere for *Water For Elephants*. My legs were like jelly as he strolled down the red carpet, and by the time he reached me I could hardly get my first question out.

'Did you manage to catch up with Charlie?' I eventually asked. His brooding brown eyes looked at me quizzically. 'I was the journo who put you in touch with him,' I explained.

After a moment the realisation dawned on him. 'Oh, was that *you* I spoke to?' he asked, his face transforming with a huge grin. 'Thanks for that—yes I'm planning to meet up with him later tonight.'

Me and R-Patz had shared a moment, and I decided then and there he was the nicest actor in Hollywood. He was such a down-to-earth, lovely guy.

Nick and I each had a celebrity 'hall pass', which we would joke about: if our favourite celebrity ever propositioned us and we accepted, it wouldn't count as cheating. Mine was R-Patz and his was Gisele Bundchen. After my second interview with Robert, Nick started to get a bit worried. 'You know the whole "hall pass" thing is a joke, right?' he muttered as we made our way into the *Water For Elephants* premiere after my chat with Robert.

'What do you mean?' I asked, stone faced. 'I'm going for a drink with Rob after the movie.'

When I saw the shock on Nick's face, I broke into a fit of giggles.

'Never, Nicky,' I said, taking his hand in mine. 'You're my only love, forever.'

◆ ◆ ◆

There have been a few instances when the image I'd held of celebrities I've admired was crushed following an interview, and funnily enough, they were all events at which Robert was present.

Reese Witherspoon—whose bubbly on-screen persona made her top my list of ultimate celebrity BFFs—was far from friendly at the premiere of *Water For Elephants*. Every answer to my question was clipped and short, and it seemed as if attending the film premiere was a total drag. I realise that some actors just want to act, and not do all the other promotional stuff, but walking a red carpet for an hour or two is really not so bad when you put things into perspective.

Another star whose off-screen persona I found to be in stark contrast to her on-screen one was Isla Fisher. In 2014,

Elle Halliwell

I attended an Australian film event in Los Angeles at which she was the star attendee alongside R-Patz, who had just filmed an Australian movie, *The Rover,* with Guy Pearce. All the Aussie media were excited to ask her about her recent roles in *The Great Gatsby* and *Bachelorette,* and her thoughts on Australia's screen talent. But she raced through the red carpet and barely had any time for the media pack, especially the print reporters, who often get the short end of the stick when it comes to celebrity red carpet chats. She gave a heartfelt speech on stage at the dinner, but the moment she finished she was overheard telling her minders she wanted to get out of there as soon as possible. 'I was supposed to have left 20 minutes ago,' I heard her tell them. Osher Günsberg was hosting a live auction at the time, offering two flights to Australia, when Isla stood up and tried to leave. 'We've got a $15,000 bid from Isla!' Osher exclaimed. Isla blanched. 'No, no!' she said, shaking her head and sitting back down again.

I was sitting at the next table and watched her conspiring with her 'people'. A few moments later she had disappeared from view, and I heard some commotion behind me. She was *crawling* between the tables towards the door! I don't know if she was trying to get some laughs but it fell flat with the crowd, who were politely watching the auction. The next morning I was interviewed by Fitzy and Wippa about the incident, and ran a story in *The Daily Telegraph.*

After the formalities I followed R-Patz out through the venue's kitchen and out a back door, thinking the on-screen vampire was leaving before I could pledge my undying love for him. Ok, I wasn't going to do that—but I hadn't been sent halfway around the world just to interview Aussie celebrities. I wanted to get a word or two from him for the paper before he left the event, so I burst through the heavy metal door, only to find him having a cigarette with a mate in the back alleyway.

'Erm, oh—the bathrooms aren't back here?' I said, looking around. My cheeks had turned a vibrant shade of pink. 'Sorry, um, enjoy your cigarettes.' I smiled at the pair, and began backing away when I heard the soft click of the kitchen door shutting. My hand reached for the door handle. There wasn't one: the door only opened from the inside! I tried to pry it open, breaking two manicured nails as I clawed it desperately, but still the door wouldn't budge. *No, no, no!* I thought, looking for another escape route.

I didn't know what to do. If I continued lurking there, R-Patz—who, despite our previous encounters, had no clue who I was—might think I was a crazy stalker trying to eavesdrop on his conversation. I slunk back out into the alleyway, looking ridiculous in my flimsy red dress, which was far too thin for the cool LA evening. R-Patz and his friend turned to me. 'It's, um—the door is, erm, locked!' I stammered, gesturing to the door. At that moment, I heard a creak as one of the kitchen hands pushed the solid door open. I was saved!

'Nice to chat R-Pat—I mean Robert, um, yeah, I'm just going to find the bathroom now,' I spluttered awkwardly. I bolted back, caught the door before it closed again and retreated into the anonymity of the two hundred-plus crowd.

By the time I'd regained my composure, I dialled my girlfriend Briana in Sydney. 'Oh my god I got to meet R-Patz again, and it was totally amazing!' I told her excitedly. 'I stalked him down a back alleyway.'

'Of course, you did, Elle,' she laughed. 'I'll let you know if a restraining order lands on your desk while you're away.'

♦ ♦ ♦

You might think that being constantly surrounded by beautiful people with seemingly perfect lives would bring all of your own insecurities to the surface. But seeing past the photoshopped portraits and carefully constructed interview responses during my time covering entertainment and fashion made me feel pretty darn good about myself.

I can't remember how many times I had to race to Myer or nearby PR agencies to borrow extra clothing items because the model, singer or actress we were shooting for Insider thought her hips/arms/legs/stomach looked fat in the samples she'd been sent.

A few years ago I worked on a cover shoot with a well-known Australian songstress, whose size-eight figure would have looked good swathed in a paper bag. During the shoot her publicist approached my editor, Kerry, the photographer and me. 'Look, for the shoot she doesn't want you to take any full-length photos of her,' the publicist said as the starlet was getting ready in the nearby change room. 'She doesn't want her legs in the shot.'

'Why, what's the problem?' the photographer asked innocently. The star's pins were slender, and hardly noticeable under the thick stockings, which she had refused to take off. 'She's just self-conscious about them,' her publicist replied.

We agreed to her request, wanting to make sure she felt relaxed so we could get a great shot.

The day before the story went to print, we also sent her our chosen cover shot for her to have a look at, even though it wasn't generally something we'd do. Her photo was cropped at the waist, and she looked stunning. A few hours later we received an email from her publicist insisting we use a different photo. 'She thinks her right eye looks a bit wonky,' the email explained.

Kerry had done the songstress a courtesy by sending the image for her reference—but it was not for her approval, as newspapers don't operate like that. The singer had been difficult throughout the shoot, and my editor was on the verge of pulling the photo completely in favour of another lesser known but much more pleasant actress.

In the end, we published our original cover shot, as well as a full-length image—legs and all—of the precious singer alongside the article.

◆ ◆ ◆

The more celebrities I dealt with, the more I realised that fame certainly wasn't all it was cracked up to be. If they were even mildly of interest to the women's gossip magazines, the paparazzi pack would do anything they could to shoot them in an unflattering light or acting inappropriately.

Photos of a beautiful TV personality walking out of the hairdresser looking glamorous would often fetch a much lower price than shots of her walking in with a bird's nest for hair and a scowl on her face.

In comparison to Sydney, however, Hollywood is in a whole new league when it comes to celebrity stalking, and The Kardashians remain the top targets.

When I first joined *The Sunday Telegraph*, Kim Kardashian was completely unknown to Australians. During a trip with Paris Hilton to Sydney in 2006, one of the paper's reporters approached Kim on Bondi Beach and asked if she could snag him an interview with Paris; he'd mistaken Kim for Paris' publicist. A year later the reality show *Keeping Up With The Kardashians* launched and catapaulted Kim and her family to the height of fame.

Witnessing the family's publicity machine in action is an impressive sight. I've interviewed Kim and Khloe a number of times, and in 2015 made a cameo appearance on an episode of *Keeping Up With The Kardashians*. I had been chosen to host the Australian launch of the family's children's clothing range, Kardashian Kids, and Khloe had flown to Sydney with a production crew to film it for the show.

Months of preparation had gone into organising the event, and Khloe's extremely large team had scheduled her visit down to the tiniest detail. Every minute was accounted for, and no element was left to chance. I had been required to wear pieces from the women's Kardashian Kollection, so about a month beforehand I went to the brand's local showroom to pick out an outfit.

Khloe and her team had already chosen what she would be wearing at the event, so my options were a carefully edited assortment of different pieces. Knowing how micromanaged the visit was, I could imagine the chaos I'd have caused if I rocked up in the same jumpsuit! Khloe's US team were so attuned to her they seemed almost psychic. I saw this firsthand during an interview with the star before the launch. She was seated opposite me and two cameras had been set up to film us. Khloe had a small TV monitor facing her, showing her face. The film crew gestured it was ready.

'So Khloe, welcome to Australia,' I began.

We started chatting, and about a minute into the interview one of Khloe's minders cut it short.

'You're not happy with the angle?' she asked Khloe. I'd seen Khloe briefly look at the monitor, but her glance had been fleeting. Sure enough, she wanted it changed. Love them or hate them, The Kardashians are a fascinating bunch.

A year prior, I had interviewed Kim Kardashian for the launch of the family's accessories range. J.Mo and I had joined The Nova Entertainment radio network a few months before. It had taken more than a year to get our show Confidential On Nova with J.Mo and Elle off the ground, but J.Mo is an incredibly determined guy. He relentlessly negotiated and eventually managed to convince the station and the News Corp powers-that-be that an entertainment show would be a huge success and a great cross-promotion opportunity for both media companies; sometimes I wonder whether J.Mo's tenaciousness simply wore them down. But four years on, our little Sunday night show has topped the ratings repeatedly in its timeslot and it's one of the highlights of our week.

Unfortunately J.Mo missed out on interviewing Kim, as he was overseas, so our producers Sophie Ainsworth and Mikey Watson invited former Miss Universe Australia Rachael Finch to fill in as co-host. Meeting Kim in the flesh was a shock. First of all she is tiny, and Rachael and I—being quite tall—towered over her, despite the crazily high heels she was sporting.

Her husband Kanye had ducked out to the shops when we arrived for the interview, which took place at Sydney's Park Hyatt hotel. Her daughter, North, was in another room with her nanny, and was a little unwell. 'Do you mind if I just go in and check on her?' Kim asked before the interview began.

We could see her team bristling, knowing a few minutes delay would throw out the entire schedule.

Rachael and I were given a choice: we could do a ten-minute interview, or an eight-minute interview and have our photo taken with her at the end. For the sake of quality journalism, we chose the former, but decided to push our luck anyway once the chat finished.

'Can we get a pic before we go?' I asked Kim directly. I saw one of her US publicists give me a death stare, but she was too late. 'Sure,' purred Kim, 'but we've got to do it in the bathroom—the light's much better.' Moments later, Rachael and I were crouching down beside the reality star, being taught how to take the perfect selfie. 'See how good the lighting is?' Kim asked us. And was right. Bathroom selfies are the way to go; just make sure not to get the toilet in the background.

I entered the media world at a very interesting time, and saw its landscape change dramatically, particularly in the showbiz sphere. These days anyone who looks half good in a bikini and can take a winning selfie gets slapped with the 'celebrity' stamp.

In the good old days before social media, anyone who had scored an Oscar, Golden Globe or Grammy nomination sat atop the celebrity importance pyramid.

To qualify for the tier below, you would have needed to have won an ARIA or Logie, or competed in an Olympic Games.

But now anyone who has walked on a runway, appeared on a reality TV show, married or had an affair with a sports star, or amassed more than 10,000 followers on Instagram qualifies as 'talent'.

And yet the A-list stars are often the least prickly to deal with. Ask a journalist who they believe is the most easygoing star in Australia, and it's likely they'll say 'Hugh Jackman'. He's an absolute pro at navigating the paparazzi. Almost every time he comes home to Oz he'll head down to Bondi, take his shirt off, jump in the water for a swim and let the city's celebrity photographers shoot to their hearts' content. He'll give them a wave, head back to his house and won't be bothered again.

At the other end of the spectrum, I can't count the number of times a WAG's representative has informed me ahead of an interview that the said wife or girlfriend won't respond to any questions involving her famous partner. In many cases, the only reason they're being interviewed is because of said partner.

One well-known wife of a certain Australian sportsman was notorious for this. Prior to hooking up with her sporty spouse, she was unknown. Soon after their engagement, however, she landed a bunch of ambassadorial roles with local fashion and beauty brands. She was a nightmare to deal with, and for a long time refused to address any questions about her private life—the only thing our readers were even vaguely interested in. Eventually media outlets got bored of her bland interviews, and the attention dropped off. It didn't take long for her to real-ise that if she wanted to become a media darling, she needed to reveal more about her life than what she put in her green breakfast smoothies.

Some stars genuinely don't want to be famous; they want to do their job, and spend the rest of their time living a low-key life away from the media spotlight, and that's fine. They are the stars who don't flirt with fellow celebrities on Twitter, who don't sell the exclusive rights to their baby shower to the gossip magazines, or go to every single event they're invited to. They know that the more boring their personal lives are seen to be, the less attention they will get from the media.

◆ ◆ ◆

Showbiz reporting can be a very thankless job, and I've had my fair share of run-ins with personalities in my time at *The Daily Telegraph*. On Melbourne Cup Day a few years back, I was in the Myer marquee at Flemington's Birdcage enclosure interviewing the brand's VIP guests. The main race had just finished and I noticed Sam Wood, from *The Bachelor*, beside me, looking pleased with himself.

'Hi Sam, my name's Elle, I'm from *The Daily Telegraph*,' I smiled. 'How did you guys go on the race? Are you having a good time?'

Sam turned to me. All of a sudden his smile turned into a sneer and his eyes narrowed. 'I'm not going to talk to you, after that story you ran yesterday.' My mind started racing as I tried to remember what yarns I'd filed the day before. They were all related to Fashions On The Field and had nothing to do with reality TV. *Had his girlfriend Snezana Markoski entered the fashion competition? Maybe I'd said something negative about her outfit?* I was quite sure I hadn't.

'Hmm, nope, I didn't write any story about you yesterday— I think you've got the wrong person,' I said, apologetically.

'It doesn't matter who wrote it, you're from *The Daily Telegraph* and you're all tarred with the same brush,' he spat, loud enough to attract stares from the racegoers beside us.

I smiled. 'Cool, no problem Sam, enjoy the rest of race day,' I said to his back as he stormed off with Snezana.

A friend who'd witnessed my dressing down had gone white. 'Are you okay, honey? That was pretty brutal,' she said, taking my hand. 'Does that happen a lot?'

'Yeah,' I laughed. 'Sometimes. I'm not fazed by that sort of stuff anymore,' I said, taking a sip of champagne. 'Let's go refill our glasses and watch the next race.'

The story Sam was referring to, I later found out, had focused on his relationship with Snezana and their plans for Christmas. Sam's beef was that the interview had been organised by a charity he was promoting and, while it got a mention online, it hadn't made the print edition.

A month or two later, I received an email from a publicist, wanting to know if I'd like to write a story about Sam Wood's new fitness app. 'I'd love to tee up a phone chat with you and Sam on Sunday,' she suggested. I was a little shocked to hear from her in light of Sam's outburst at me and my fellow *Telegraph* journalists.

I giggled, and politely declined.

◆ ◆ ◆

In 2013, almost three years after the launch of the 'J.Mo and Elle' column, Breenie announced his resignation from *The Sunday Telegraph*. His departure was the beginning of a huge change for News Limited's editorial department, which included the amalgamation of the *Daily Telegraph* and *Sunday Telegraph*'s editorial teams. We were to operate on a seven-day roster, with only a few reporters remaining as dedicated staff for the Sunday edition. 'J.Mo and Elle' was rebranded as 'Sydney Confidential', and despite having competed against *The Daily Telegraph*'s gossip team for stories and paparazzi photos for years, we were now obliged to share the love and work as a team. It took some adjusting.

The move, however, proved the perfect opportunity for me to move back into a more fashion-focused role, and eventually I took over the Fashion Confidential page on Saturdays, contributing fashion stories to *The Daily Telegraph*'s general news pages, and picture spreads in the Saturday edition.

By this point I'd amassed years of experience in the fashion space, and the impostor syndrome I'd battled with at the start of my fashion reporting tenure had faded in favour of self-assurance and confidence in my ability to write bravely and honestly about designers and the industry in general.

My reporting style didn't sit too well with some of the country's fashion folk. I had no qualms about calling a designer out if the courts had found they hadn't paid their suppliers or manufacturers. Being such a small industry, it's common for our designers to be treated like rock stars if they draw praise internationally. We have some incredibly creative designers, but I've come to realise that while many are ridiculously talented at creating beautiful clothing, just as many are completely clueless about how to successfully run a business. If you look at some of Australia's most successful labels, you'll often find they are headed by a duo, with one focused on the design, and another handling the growth of the business; Camilla and Marc, Bassike, Ginger & Smart and Zimmermann are just a few.

The global financial crisis saw the demise of an unprecedented number of well-known Australian designer brands including Lisa Ho, Kirrily Johnston, Ksubi and Bettina Liano, which all fell into the hands of administrators. Their woes made headlines around the country, but what didn't receive much publicity was the effect it had on the Australian garment industry's outworkers—the pattern makers and suppliers who also lost out as a result.

Over the years I've received countless calls from individual contractors claiming they hadn't been paid by a top Aussie designer for work done. Often the sum was too small to warrant court action, but after a while a lost $1000 here and another $2000 there can quickly add up and cause a lot of financial strain. Many have told me they continue working with the same designers for fear they will otherwise go offshore, and there won't be enough work to support the already strained local textile and clothing manufacturing industry.

While writing about fashion isn't saving the world, I took comfort in knowing I was helping to keep designers accountable and giving a voice to the uncelebrated identities of Australia's fashion industry.

My job wasn't all about covering badly behaving designers; I'd often be invited to preview fashion and accessory collections to find pieces to feature in the paper's fashion spreads. Sometimes these would be a major affair, replete with a runway show and cocktails or lunch; other times it was just a quick viewing at the designer's studio.

In late 2015, I was invited to view a new collection from an Australian jewellery label. In a fun twist, the designer had hired a tarot reader to give readings to the stylists and fashion editors who came to see the new range. I had little faith in clairvoyants. I'd had a reading done once at a Mind, Body, Spirit festival and had been told that I'd travel in my twenties and would have a few children. It was hardly a revelation. But Tuesdays were quiet, so I put my name down.

The clairvoyant, a woman in her early fifties, was softly spoken and dressed in a handmade red patchwork jacket. Her warm, open smile put me at ease as I shuffled the tarot cards in front of me. 'Your grandmother isn't well,' she said, looking down at the spread my hands had chosen. My grandmother had, in fact, broken her hip at the time, and was not in a good way. She was in her early nineties, and I'd been told that many people didn't recover well from such injuries so late in life. 'Don't worry; she's going to be fine,' the clairvoyant said, noticing my reaction. She spoke further about my work and some unimportant things, and then towards the end of the reading she took my right hand. She turned my palm up and studied its lines as intently as a hiker reading a map.

'Hmm,' she said eventually. 'How's your health?'

'Fine,' I replied. I was one of those people who took mere seconds to fill out forms at health spas, simply ticking 'no' to allergies, medications, sensitivities and prior medical conditions. Aside from the odd cold and throat infection on holidays, and of course my chronic anxiety, I was fine.

'So, no major health problems—nothing like that?' she asked again.

At this point I was starting to get a bit miffed. *Do I look sick?* I thought to myself. I'd done my makeup that morning, and with my current diet of whatever I felt like eating at the time, I looked far from malnourished.

'No, seriously, never had any serious health problems. Why are you asking?'

'There's quite a noticeable break in your health line,' she said, pointing to the curved line which ended at my wrist. 'If I were you I'd keep an eye on your health over the next year or two.'

She looked me in the eye. 'I see a few years of illness, so just monitor it.'

A few weeks later I spoke to my dad, and asked about Granny. 'They've taken her off the morphine and the pain drugs and she's doing great,' he said. 'She's reading the paper, getting angry at the nurses, and is back up and walking around.'

I was so relieved, but had already forgotten about the clairvoyant and her other predictions.

The Search Begins

May 2016

The moment we came home from our consultation at the Lifehouse, we began our search for another woman who had been pregnant while battling chronic myeloid leukaemia, or CML. I signed up to a bunch of online forums, and scanned through posts tagged with the words 'pregnancy' or 'baby'. Discussions about stopping medication in order to try for a baby were common, but I found zero mention of being diagnosed with chronic leukaemia *and* being pregnant.

Nick called the Leukaemia Foundation that afternoon to ask if anyone else in their database had been diagnosed with CML early on in her pregnancy. If so, perhaps we could call them to gain a little more insight into the challenge we were facing?

Since 'D-Day' I had noticed an incredible change in my normally easily distracted husband. The exhausting emotional rollercoaster had left me sedate and distracted; Nick, however, was wired. He had developed a level of focus I hadn't seen in him before, and began spending hours on his computer, trying to find information on my illness and a precedent for our situation.

Even Doc had been impressed with Nick's determination.

A few days after our meeting with the Prof, Doc rang to ask how I was doing. Nick began explaining the details of my cancer and how advanced it was, rattling off terms like 'Sokal score', 'BCR–ABL' and 'Philadelphia chromosome'. He then delved into details of the research he had been doing regarding CML and pregnancy.

'Mate, I've got no idea what you're talking about,' laughed Doc, 'but it sounds like you're close to discovering Lorenzo's Oil, so keep at it!'

'Basically,' Nick continued, 'Prof said the safest option is to end the pregnancy, freeze Elle's eggs and start the drugs. But we'll have to wait another month to abort the pregnancy, then who knows how long until Elle gets her period again? That could take another month or two, and then we could be in September by the time she's finished all that and can start taking the tyrosine kinase inhibitors,' Nick said.

'That's only a couple of months before she's due, then,' Doc said slowly, his crazily intelligent mind whirring away. 'And there's always the option of inducing her early if it looks like the cancer's progressing quickly. Premature babies have pretty good outlooks these days. Look, it's something to think about, but just take your time. You've still got a few weeks until Elle really has to decide.'

The Leukaemia Foundation was incredibly helpful when Nick called. I was still unable to make phone calls to anyone bar family. The more I spoke about it, the more vivid my situation became, and I wasn't yet ready to face that level of reality.

Melissa, a patient coordinator at the Foundation, promised to post out an information pack, and signed me up to its Blood Buddies program, which aims to connect newly diagnosed leukaemia patients with others who had faced similar circumstances, as a way to provide emotional support.

'I'm going to need some time to work out if there's anyone who might have been in a similar situation,' she eventually told Nick. 'In the meantime, let me know if you and your wife need any assistance in the way of transport to and from appointments, or information on support services.'

If nobody else in Australia had been through this, perhaps we needed to expand our search. I signed up to an international organisation called Hope For Two, which connected women who had been diagnosed with cancer while pregnant. Breast, skin and bowel cancer were common in the women's stories, but not CML. I emailed the organisation, explaining my situation, and asking if they knew of anyone with a similar story to mine.

Now I had to wait.

I shut down my laptop, flopped on the couch and let TV presenter Maeve O'Meara distract me from thoughts of my upcoming biopsy with a Korean cooking *Food Safari*.

Drilling Down

It may span just over three months, but ask a new mum how long her first trimester of pregnancy felt and most will say much longer than that, for so many reasons. First, there is the worry over whether or not the pregnancy will stick; every trip to the toilet involving the holding of breath until you can stand up and check the bowl isn't specked with red. Red, the colour of danger, the symbol of 'stop'.

Then there's the at-times unbearable nausea, which can be triggered by anything from a work colleague's egg salad to the collective whiff of post-work armpits keeping you company on the evening bus commute.

But patiently waiting to explain the reason for your newfound obsession with empire-line frocks and cheese, honey and pickle sandwiches to friends can be excruciating.

For Nick and me, telling loved ones about our surprise pregnancy was something we were happy to postpone. We had already broken tragic news; we didn't want to have to deal another blow, at least so soon.

But having nobody else to talk to but each other was extremely isolating. I wanted to unload all of my feelings—my fears, my sorrows, my pain—onto someone else, to share the uncertainty, to be comforted and be told that I would—no, *we* would—be ok.

But I had to hold my tongue. I had to lie.

'When do you start treatment?' friends would inevitably ask when I told them about the cancer.

'I'm not sure; I have to discuss fertility options first. But fill me in on what's happening in the land of the living,' I'd say brightly, trying to direct the conversation away from tricky questions. And my answer wasn't completely untrue. At that stage, terminating the pregnancy and freezing my eggs was the most reasonable, sane choice. It would enable me to begin attacking my leukaemia within a couple of months, and I'd have a backup plan if the proposed treatment affected my reproductive system, which was a possibility. I would have to be on the drugs for at least five years before we could even consider trying for a baby, according to Prof. By this time I would be 36. It wasn't exactly old, but it would technically put me in the category of 'geriatric mother'. I had fallen pregnant easily this time, but had no idea whether that was just a fluke. Would I be able to fall pregnant in five or six years time? Would I still even be *alive* in five years time?

I had so many questions myself that I was hardly in a position to answer any from well-meaning friends.

◆ ◆ ◆

Telling our parents was nerve-racking. Until now, it had just been me and Nick trying to figure out how to make the right choice. But our families would have their own views and opinions, and I was worried it would confuse the situation even more. Would they call me insane for even considering keeping the baby? Would they think I was insane *not* to?

We really had no choice but to tell them, though, as the constant questions about what date my treatment would start were getting harder and harder to sidestep. We would tell friends later, but we had to spill the beans to our folks.

'So, we've got some news,' Nick said. We were sitting opposite his parents in their living room, as well as my mum. 'Yes, some more news.'

I could see them trying to figure out what could possibly be worthy of a family sit-down less than a week after the revelation I had an incurable blood cancer.

'It's a bit of a complication. Elle's pregnant.'

'Congratulations!' Nick's mother Het exclaimed—then checked her excitement momentarily when she saw our grim faces.

'Look, we don't know what we're going to do at this point, but obviously it makes things very complicated, and that's why I haven't been able to start treatment yet,' I explained, keeping my voice level.

Mum had brought her hands to her mouth and hadn't uttered a word.

'On Wednesday we're going down to Adelaide to meet with another doctor—he's a world expert in CML—to get a bit more of an idea about what we should do. The Prof said the safest way would be to terminate, but we wanted to get another opinion before making a decision.'

They were all silent for a moment.

'Well,' Nick's father Pete finally said. 'Whatever you decide, we're here for you—and we know you'll make the right choice, whatever that is.'

Dad's reaction was less tactful. 'I think you should keep the baby,' he declared, shortly after I broke the news to him over the phone that afternoon. I was shocked and upset at what I believed was his obvious disregard for my own safety, but I later came to realise his blunt opinion had been influenced by that fateful week at Woody Head, when he and Mum had been faced with the same decision.

◆ ◆ ◆

The biopsy would confirm I did indeed have the Philadelphia chromosome, the definitive marker of chronic myeloid leukaemia. Two scientists, Peter Nowell and David Hungerford, discovered the Philadelphia Chromosome in 1959, when they noticed that the DNA of the CML patients they tested was abnormal. In 1971 another scientist, Janet Rowley, discovered the abnormality was caused when pieces of chromosomes 9 and 22 broke apart and attached to each other. Nobody knows exactly what causes this to happen, and why no other cancer exhibits this same chromosome switch.

I'd read on a few online forums that the biopsy procedure was a very unpleasant experience. I'm no chicken when it comes to pain, but the idea of having my hip bone punctured by a giant needle didn't sound very appealing.

Nick and I arrived at the Royal Prince Alfred the morning of the operation and, after filling out a ream of medical forms, I was called into a consultation room to prepare for the procedure. A nurse explained that I would be drowsy from the sedatives, so I would be required to spend a while in the recovery room afterwards.

'Just to let you know, I'm pregnant,' I told the nurse. I also explained I was taking blood-thinning medication to prevent my now prolific platelets from causing a blood clot.

'Right, ok, I'll make sure the doctors know this,' she replied, scribbling notes on my form.

I slipped out of my clothes—a chic, military-green knit sweater and matching skirt I'd bought from Melbourne fashion label Scanlan Theodore to wear at fashion week— and into my white hospital gown, in a small changing room. *If I'm going to take on cancer*, I thought to myself as I got dressed that morning, *I'm not going to do it looking like a dag.*

I didn't mind the white cotton hospital gown. A kimono-style waist belt would add some shape, I mused, cinching it with my hands and doing a turn in the mirrored room, as if trying on a frock for the races. *If only.* I took a selfie, my mouth in a lopsided grin, and sent it to Briana. She had taken the news badly, and I hoped the photo would show her I hadn't completely fallen apart. I'd even put on makeup.

After stepping out in my shapeless hospital frock, a nurse directed me to a crisp white-sheeted bed and swabbed my inner arm with an alcohol wipe. After a few failed painful attempts, the nurse finally found a suitable vein for the cannula, which would deliver the sedatives.

The doctor in charge of the biopsy came into the room a few minutes later. 'I've got some bad news,' he said, looking at the cannula sticking out of my right arm. 'Because you're pregnant, we're going to have to perform the biopsy without the general anaesthetic.'

I let out the breath I had been holding as he spoke. Maybe it couldn't be that painful, I thought, if they offered the operation without sedatives.

'It's not that bad,' he said, with a reassuring pat on my arm. 'An elderly man before you had it done without the anaesthetic, and he's fine. Your husband can come in and hold your hand during the procedure.'

'Ok, whatever is safest for the baby,' I said. 'Can I get this thing out of my arm then?' I asked, pointing to the empty cannula.

'No, we'll keep it in there, just in case.' *Bugger.*

I had two doctors overseeing the procedure. Both were slight of frame and appeared to be in their late thirties. 'Ok, Ms Halliwell, first we're going to turn you on your side and give you a local anaesthetic,' one of them explained. He then presented me with a very large metal needle, attached to what looked like the top of an oversized corkscrew. 'Then we're going to push this into your hip bone to take a sample of your bone marrow. You'll feel a pushing sensation. It usually takes about half an hour—but it depends how strong your bones are,' he said, giving me a wry smile.

Even with the local anaesthetic, the pain was excruciating. As the doctor pushed the needle through the thin flesh of my hip and hit my bone, sharp pains shot down my entire left femur. It was the strangest sensation, like someone was scratching against my skeleton with a knife. About thirty minutes in, the doctor was sweating as my bone refused to give way to the needle.

'You do have very hard bones,' he joked. 'You must drink a lot of milk.'

By this point, I wasn't in the mood for humour. Nick and the nurse were trying in vain to distract me from all the action as the doctors continued to work on my stubborn hip, which refused to give up its tender marrow.

'How long have you two been married?' the nurse asked me.

'Almost. Three. Years,' I said through gritted teeth, tears streaming down my face. Nick had started getting pins and needles in one of his hands due to the grip I had maintained on his wrist.

Suddenly I felt the bone give way and the rod crunch through my bone marrow.

'We got it!' said the doctor, wiping drops of sweat from his brow.

I thought I was going to pass out from the prolonged pain, which had worked its way down my leg, but slowly as I relaxed my tense muscles the pain became more tolerable. I could finally rest.

A short while later, I heard the two doctors conversing quietly in the corner of the room. I could hear a *Bang! Bang!* as one of them hit something against the ceramic basin against the wall. There was a pause, and a long sigh. 'I can't get it out,' I heard one of them say, quietly.

The same doctor walked over to me, looking sheepish. 'I'm really sorry, but your bones were so hard the needle has bent and we can't get the marrow out. We're going to have to take another sample.'

At that moment I began to sob. I had spent the past fortnight trying to keep myself emotionally together, but the thirty minutes of uninterrupted agony was more than my brain could handle.

I nodded my consent. I was too distressed to talk and my jaw was trembling, but I knew I had no choice but to continue.

The physical pain had suddenly turned my illness from a theory—a flimsy monochrome possibility—into a technicolour, concrete reality.

I felt beaten as I sat afterwards in the padded, oversized blue chair in the recovery room for almost four hours—much longer than usual due to excess bleeding from my blood-thinning drugs. The holes in my back weren't clotting up, and nurses had to keep changing my bandages. I hadn't brought much in the way of warm layers, and the room was blisteringly cold. I was also light-headed from hunger. The nurse pointed to a small kitchen. 'You can get a cup of tea and something to eat while you wait to be discharged,' she said.

I went over to check out the options. There was a tower of Styrofoam cups and plastic spoons beside the boiling water dispenser, and a big plastic tub of teabags and sugar sachets. I cringed. My diagnosis had ignited in me an acute phobia of chemicals, processed foods, medicines and plastic packaging.

Six months prior, I had no more than a mild awareness of the hundreds of toxins I was coming into contact with each day via cosmetics, cleaning products, food packaging and even seemingly innocuous tax receipts.

I'd refined my diet in my late twenties by tweaking certain eating and drinking habits slowly, which had ensured the changes lasted. Over a period of about three years my coffee order had evolved from a strong cappuccino with three teaspoons of sugar to a flat white with half a teaspoon. My once-regular soft drink consumption was also eventually eliminated in favour of filtered water, and I now rarely drank anything from a can, unless it was a special occasion.

While looking into fertility diets I had also discovered the importance of the body's gut microbiome, and how to nourish it with the right fuel in the form of prebiotic vegetables and fermented foods like sauerkraut and kefir.

But I couldn't have predicted the seismic shift which occurred in my thinking when I was faced with my own mortality. I suddenly realised I could no longer remain in blissful ignorance of the impact my modern diet and lifestyle had had on my health, and what effects it could have on my unborn child.

I considered having a black tea, then instantly imagined the boiling water reacting with the polystyrene, turning the liquid into a cancerous cocktail which would invade my already traumatised blood cells with each sip. I looked for ceramic mugs. None. Anyway, they would have been washed with toxic antibacterial dish soap, I decided. I didn't even want to drink a cup of water from the white squeaky cups, even though my body was screaming for some. I checked the fridge for something to eat, maybe a piece of fruit or a nut bar. All I found were two dozen packaged sandwiches, each pair of doughy, white slices encasing a golden yellow strip. It could have been butter. No, judging by the fluffy texture it was probably margarine, plus maybe a slice of processed cheese.

I looked behind me into the recovery room. An elderly woman sat in her blue chair opposite me wearing the same white cotton ensemble and munching on one half of a calorie-laden but nutrient-bare sandwich. Her bare skinny legs were covered in varicose veins, her feet swathed in a pair of navy sheepskin slippers that looked so comfortable I was tempted to wrestle them from her. Another young woman sat a few seats away, eating a cookie and sipping something hot from one of the white foam cups. Weren't all the people in this hospital room sick, or at least possibly sick? A square of refined white flour filled with preservatives was the last thing any of us needed. *We should do a push at The Daily Telegraph to run a campaign for better hospital food,* I thought. *Maybe we can get Jamie Oliver on board. A roast vegetable and quinoa salad would be a good addition to that sad, vitamin-deficient fridge. Maybe with a green smoothie or acai bowl option?*

The next time I had to spend any time in hospital, I vowed to bring my own little cooler bag of wholefoods, and my own ceramic mug.

◆ ◆ ◆

Waiting for the biopsy results was brutal—as mentally agonising as the procedure had been physically. A tide of nausea had begun to rise in my gut. I wasn't sure if it was the beginnings of first trimester morning sickness, or my anxiousness to know the outcome of this latest test. My specialist had stressed that there was very little doubt I had CML. The biopsy was simply to get more information about the leukaemia, and detect any mutations that could complicate my treatment.

But despite the Prof's confidence in his diagnosis, I had managed to almost convince myself the test would show otherwise. It would end my nightmare: I'd be told there'd been a terrible mistake and there was actually no sign of leukaemic cells in my bone marrow. I'd utter a cry of relief and Nick and I would slowly get back to our normal lives. All that would remain from our ordeal would be a compelling story to share around the dinner table with new friends at parties. 'Before I start, let me assure you this has a happy ending,' Nick would tell them, before delving into the events of 2016. 'But you'll never believe what happened before we found out we were having "Junior".'

Nick was still coming to grips with our situation at this point, but his positive attitude had for the most part returned and it proved a welcome distraction during my recovery.

Doc called to check on me post-op. My lower back was tender, but aside from a bit of discomfort and fatigue I was feeling ok. 'We'll need to arrange an ultrasound for the pregnancy,' Doc said. He would book it in for about three weeks time, to confirm I was definitely pregnant and the embryo was viable. I had taken about half a dozen more tests since the first. They were piling up in a clear zip-lock bag, which I kept in a plastic tub above my fridge. I would check them periodically, laying them out side by side in order of date. May 1—the pricey Clearblue test—still said *Pregnant, 3–4 weeks*. The rest were small, no-frills ones I'd taken from Doc's clinic, displaying two red lines for a positive result. Each day the telltale lines had grown darker as the level of pregnancy hormones had risen in my body.

It became almost a morning ritual. I'd wake up, grab a test on my way to the toilet and pee on it. I'd hold my breath, still unsure as to how I would feel if the matching line was lighter, or absent. Life would be a little less complicated, and I'd just be sick, not sick and pregnant.

But each time I saw the second line appear in the positive test window, I felt a pang of relief, and wonder.

Adelaide

'Shelley Bell!' Nick exclaimed, breaking me out of my daytime TV-induced stupor. In the days following the biopsy I had struggled to find the motivation to do much of anything. Showering, once a pleasure, felt like a punishment, forcing me to sit with my own thoughts in a glass cage, the water failing to wash away the only thing I wanted it to.

But an hour of infomercials and half of a midday movie was both distracting and boring enough to put me into a restless sleep, and it had become my new daily ritual.

Shelley Bell. The name reminded me of my own. *Shell and*

Elle. Shell Bell. Elle Belle had been my nickname for as long as I could remember. Sometimes it was Ella Bella, or Ellie Bellie.

But Shelley Bell and I shared much more than similar-sounding names.

Nick repeated the name again, this time with more urgency. He walked over to me, took my hands in his and pulled me off the couch without giving me time to protest. 'I found this woman named Shelley Bell who I think went through the same thing as we are,' he said, his eyes wide with excitement as he dragged me towards his office desk.

He gestured to an article splashed across his computer monitor. It was the front page of the Leukaemia Foundation's Spring 2008 newsletter. 'Healthy baby born to Perth mum diagnosed with CML during pregnancy,' the headline read, beside a head-shot of an attractive woman smiling with a swaddled newborn in her arms.

'It's not exactly what happened to us,' Nick said, 'but it's pretty close, and I reckon it's worth trying to track her down.'

I read through the article, hope growing in my belly with each line I devoured. According to the newsletter, the mum-of-three had been diagnosed with chronic myeloid leukaemia that year while pregnant with her fourth child. She had been put on interferon for the duration of the pregnancy, which kept her cancer under control until she could begin taking the relatively new drug, Glivec, once the baby was born.

'She went off the interferon for a couple of days before the birth, to build up her strength, and Amelie was born on June 3,' the article read. '"She was born so healthy and against the odds," said Shelley who began taking Glivec the following day.'

Healthy.

A healthy baby girl. I felt as though a rope had suddenly dropped into the dark well I had been trapped in. Someone else was out there who had felt the same pain. She had faced a similar choice to the one I would soon be forced to make. A smile worked its way across my face, and I turned towards Nick. It was the first I'd given him in more than a week, and he returned it with an even bigger grin. I could see how proud he was of himself.

'You'd make a pretty good investigatory journalist, Nicky,' I said. I wrapped my arms around his neck and quietly sobbed.

I had so many questions.

Shelley's daughter would be almost eight years old by now, I calculated. I had no idea what had happened to her since the article had been published. Had these miracle new CML drugs worked to suppress her cancer? Was she still alive? Would she be willing to speak to me about her ordeal?

Nick called the Leukaemia Foundation. 'Hi Melissa, I tracked down one of your old newsletters and found a woman from Perth who was also pregnant and had CML,' he explained. 'Her name's Shelley Bell. We were wondering if you had any contact information for her and would mind reaching out to see if she would talk to us.'

◆ ◆ ◆

'We've managed to track Shelley down,' Melissa told us a few days later. I felt giddy, a mix of nerves, excitement and trepidation fighting for my attention.

She paused. 'I explained your situation to Shelley, and while I know you're very keen to speak to her, we both feel it's best to wait until you've made your decision independently about the pregnancy first. It's a very personal choice and I don't think she wants to influence your decision either way.'

My elevated mood deflated instantly, but I put myself in Shelley's shoes and could understand her reasoning. It was too much to ask of a stranger, to dump the weight of responsibility in her hands. If I died, or became too sick to carry my baby to full term, she shouldn't have to feel responsible for influencing my decision.

It was a choice I had to make myself. I had to own it, and prepare for whatever outcome it led me to.

◆ ◆ ◆

A fortnight after my earth-shattering leukaemia diagnosis, I still hadn't returned to work. I had emailed Mick Carroll, my editor, a couple of hours after finding out, because it was just two days before Insider was due to go to print, and I was worried I'd be leaving him in the lurch.

Hey Mick,

I got some bad news today from my doctor. Really bad news. I've got leukaemia. I am hoping to take some time off work just to find out my treatment options and come to terms with it. I feel really bad about abandoning Insider, apologies for this.

Also, you're the only person I've told so far.

Speak soon,

E

I'd put my hand up to edit Insider, the showbiz section, while a replacement was found for its previous editor, who was moving interstate. I really wanted to impress Mick and show him I could handle the responsibility of editing such a well-read, popular section. Mick was Breenie's successor, and had been editor at *The Sunday Telegraph* since 2012. He was no pushover, and knew exactly what he wanted from his reporters to put out the best Sunday paper possible, but he was a very fair boss and had a heart of gold. He assured me I could take as much time as I needed, and to keep him across any more news as I received it.

When I wrote the email, the gravity of my illness clearly hadn't fully registered in my brain. I was more concerned about missing work the next day than the fact I had an incurable blood cancer. Unfortunately, my promotion to 'acting section editor' had begun just four days before my diagnosis. If the universe believed my destiny lay elsewhere than editing a liftout, surely, I mused, it could have found a less dramatic way to nudge me in a different direction than slapping me with leukaemia.

◆ ◆ ◆

I was convinced we'd be stuck in the lift as it shuddered up towards the floor of our hotel room. The bargain accommodation I'd booked was on the outskirts of Adelaide and in dire need of upkeep, especially its elevators. Neither of us had been to South Australia before—a state known for its rolling vine-covered hills and emerging food scene—but our first impression was very underwhelming, thanks to the room I'd booked online—the cheapest I could find—for our meeting the next day with CML specialist Professor Tim Hughes.

After an agonising few minutes, the ancient lift creaked open into a dreary hallway and we rolled our suitcases along the thread-bare green carpet to our room. The pokey little space felt cold, and I shuddered. I was exhausted from the flight and my back was still aching from yesterday's biopsy. I was desperately looking forward to a long, hot bath or shower and an afternoon kip.

'Where the *hell* did you find this place, Elle?' Nick asked as he scanned the dilapidated room. The heavy beige curtains had begun to fade around their edges and were swaying from the icy breeze blowing through the poorly sealed windowpanes. An aroma of mould and artificial air freshener was wafting from the pink-tiled bathroom, and the knob for the ancient air-conditioner had fallen off.

'The photos I saw looked fine,' I mumbled. 'But yeah, they must have been taken in the 80s . . . I probably should've looked around a bit more.'

Finding another place to stay was out of the question. We still didn't know what my illness meant for us financially, and we'd already spent more than we would've liked on the last-minute flights.

'It'll be fine honey, it's only for one night,' I reassured him, trying to sound positive.

I opened a small wardrobe beside the bathroom and found a thick, green blanket on the top shelf. After inspecting it for any questionable stains I wrapped it around my shivering shoulders and collapsed on the bed, where I quickly fell into a dreamless sleep.

The next morning we caught a taxi to Rundle Mall for some breakfast before our appointment. Eating out had become a problem for me, as I refused to eat anything that looked even remotely processed. We walked for about two kilometres looking for a cafe serving organic, or at least free-range, eggs and green juices. After about an hour we found a tiny hole-in-the wall coffee shop that fit the bill.

I ordered poached eggs with avocado on gluten-free toast. The eggs tasted like small white balls of heaven, and the avocado was dusted with sea salt and chilli flakes and set my tastebuds dancing. 'Oh, my, god . . . this is . . . the best breakfast . . . I've ever eaten,' I said in between delicious mouthfuls.

Nick reminded me that I said the exact same thing about Sunday's breakfast. And Saturday's. Every meal I ate while pregnant tasted like it had been laced with monosodium glutamate—the flavour just seemed enhanced and I couldn't get enough of it.

'What do you think he's going to say?' I asked Nick as we left the cafe, our bellies sated.

'If he says it's completely stupid of us to keep the baby, then I think you really need to consider getting on the drugs straight away,' he replied. 'He's going to know more about it than any other doctor, so we'll just have to wait and see what he recommends.'

I put my arm around his and leaned on his shoulder as we waited to cross the road at North Terrace.

'I feel sick, I'm so nervous,' I said. 'It might have been all the food I ate, too, but I am *really* nervous.'

We met Professor Hughes at his clinic at the Royal Adelaide Hospital's Department of Haematology. He was a kind-looking man in his fifties, and made us feel comfortable from the moment we walked in.

Prof Hughes was the Head of Translational Leukaemia Research at the South Australian Health and Medical Research Institute and had published more than 100 articles in peer-reviewed journals relating to blood disorders, including chronic myeloid leukaemia. Before our arrival we had emailed him a detailed summary of my condition and our current predicament, and he had been liaising with Prof since I'd been diagnosed.

'At the moment what we think you're dealing with is chronic-phase CML. And the Sokal score is low,' he explained.

The Sokal index was developed by Joseph E. Sokal before the introduction of the new tyrosine kinase inhibitor drugs as a way of determining the prognosis of CML patients. A Sokal score of below 0.8 is considered low, suggesting my illness had been diagnosed in its infancy.

'Do you know of anyone who has been in my situation before and has carried a baby?' I asked.

He shook his head. 'No I don't. Of my patients, there was one in a similar situation, but she decided to terminate, and she's now currently in treatment-free remission and doing very well.'

I swallowed. It was not the answer I was hoping for.

'Look, if you decide to proceed with the pregnancy there are two risks,' Professor Hughes continued. 'One is that the disease can go into blast crisis, and that's something which we can't always predict very well. The second risk is whether having that delay over the nine months will have an impact on your chances of being able to eventually stop taking the drugs at some point.'

Nick mentioned the possible use of interferon if we decided to risk keeping the pregnancy. We'd been told the drug did not cross the placenta, and studies had shown the injections were relatively safe during the later stages of pregnancy.

'It's not an easy drug to tolerate,' Professor Hughes admitted. 'I've had a lot of experience of treating people with interferon and it's really tough. You get fatigued, depressed, and it can really impact your quality of life.'

My despondency was increasing with every word he spoke.

'The time of maximum risk for you, Elle, is the next 12 months,' he said bluntly. 'Once we get this disease down to below 1 per cent in your blood and bone marrow, we know your risk of progression is getting very low—but it's not zero now, and it won't be until we get it down to that point.'

Our faces were now much less hopeful-looking than when we'd first walked in.

'What way were you leaning?' he asked, even though I knew he already knew our answer.

Nick looked at me, and saw my almost imperceptible nod. 'We think we wanted to keep it,' he said eventually.

'I understand that,' Professor Hughes replied softly. 'While you can never give guarantees, the chances are really good. As long as you accept that there *is* a risk—and we can modify that to some degree with interferon during pregnancy. It's going to be a tough time for you, but the dose would be modified for you to be able to continue with the pregnancy—then I would say as soon as you deliver . . . the sooner you start on the tyrosine kinase inhibitors, the better.'

Our Tiger Air flight out of Adelaide was delayed, giving us plenty of time to absorb everything we'd heard.

Nick took my hands as we sat in the departure lounge. I could barely keep my eyes open and my body had started to ache again from the biopsy wound.

'Look, Elle,' he said, his voice low and serious. 'From what Professor Hughes said there is a risk. And considering you were unlucky enough to be that one in 100,000 to get CML, a one in 20 risk that this could go very pear-shaped is high enough to worry about. Plus if you go ahead with the pregnancy, you might never reach full remission. *You* have to be the main priority right now.'

145

Elle Halliwell

'I've made up my mind already,' I whispered. My eyelids were fighting to stay open as I sat slumped on the uncomfortable departure gate seat. I leaned against Nick's shoulder.

'If the ultrasound shows a heartbeat, we're keeping this baby.'

24 May 2016

Dear baby,

I saw you today, for the very first time. You looked like a little peanut; a tiny, 1.14 cm peanut. I heard your heart beating, super fast, and wondered if that was normal. 'Yep, that's exactly what we expect to see,' the sonographer said as she rubbed my small belly with a cold gel-covered probe. 'It all looks good, there's a strong, clear heartbeat.' Her words made me sob and laugh at the same time. Your dad cried, too, but he said he got some dust in his eyes. You'll like him. He's pretty funny.

I didn't think I'd see your little heart beating on that monitor. I thought you would have decided life with a sick mum wasn't for you, and there would be nothing but a hollowness where you had once existed for just a few weeks. Seven weeks and one day, the sonographer said. You don't know it yet, but you've already made your mark on Earth. You've turned a self-centred, materialistic workaholic into someone more worthy of being your mum. Someone who would move mountains to keep you safe and thriving. I've been reading heaps of books on how to keep you healthy. I hope the prenatal vitamins don't taste as bad to you as they do to me, and I think you're going to like oranges as I can't seem to get enough of them these days. I've become quite obsessed with food in general so I think you're going to have a healthy appetite.

It's a little bit early as I don't think you'll have ears for another few months, but I created a playlist of songs for you which I listen to every morning when I wake up. Most of them are upbeat, like Bobby McFerrin's 'Don't Worry, Be Happy' and 'I got You Babe', by Sonny and Cher, but some of them, like Roberta Flack's 'The First Time Ever I Saw Your Face', make me cry. I've even got a few Disney classics on there, like the theme song to Beauty and The Beast, *which I loved as a child.*

I can't promise that we will get to meet each other. We have a long way to go, and so much could happen.

But I promise I'm going to do whatever it takes to get us there, because I already know I need you, and love you.

Mum

'Hi Elle, my name's Shelley and I've been given your number from the Leukaemia Foundation. I'm really sorry to hear that you have CML too. It must have been such a shock and I know it's a really scary time for you right now. But also congratulations on your pregnancy!'

I had received the text message from Shelley a few days after making our decision to keep the baby. Shelley was a mum of three from Perth, and had been diagnosed after having a blood test early in her pregnancy eight years ago.

My voice cracked when she answered the phone. She was the first person I had spoken to who not only had CML, but had gone through what I was in the middle of dealing with. The void of loneliness I was in became a little bit smaller at that moment.

'How are you doing?' I asked. Shelley replied that she was doing well, as was her daughter, Amelie, with whom she had been pregnant when she was diagnosed.

She explained she had taken interferon during the pregnancy. 'It was rough,' she added. 'I'd take it every second day and that day I felt too sick to eat or do much of anything. The days I didn't take it I felt ok, but I lost a lot of weight and I did worry that the baby wasn't going to get enough nutrition, but my mum is a nurse and said babies were designed to take what they needed from their mothers first, so not to worry. And she was born healthy.'

I wanted to reach into the phone and hug her. If she had a happy ending, perhaps there was a chance for us, too.

◆ ◆ ◆

'Now Prof, are you *sure* she's got it?' Nick asked as we sat in the white clinic room.

'Yes, I'm pretty sure,' replied Prof confidently. He pulled up the results from the biopsy. 'An abnormal clone was detected that showed the Philadelphia translocation. That's absolutely stock-standard chronic myeloid leukaemia.'

'That's good,' I sighed.

Strangely, I felt relief. It's not like Prof had said I didn't have cancer—but the fact I didn't have a more complicated cancer was a weight off my mind.

Prof had more good news for us. As a result of his previous experience with interferon use in young women who were pregnant and who were also suffering from other bone marrow disorders closely related to CML, he had successfully persuaded the hospital's Drug Committee to allow him to treat them with a slow-release, or pegylated, form of interferon during their pregnancies. Prof told me I was also eligible to be treated with this type of interferon which had fewer side effects and only had to be injected once a week.

Despite its use in pregnant women with multiple sclerosis and a number of other illnesses, pegylated interferon is a category B3 drug, which the Therapeutic Goods Administration describes as:

> Drugs which have been taken by only a limited number of pregnant women and women of childbearing age, without an increase in the frequency of malformation or other direct or indirect harmful effects on the human fetus having been observed.
>
> Studies in animals have shown evidence of an increased occurrence of fetal damage, the significance of which is considered uncertain in humans.

It wasn't ideal, but it was much safer than the tyrosine kinase inhibitors, which were category D and highly suspected of causing foetal damage.

◆ ◆ ◆

Shelley had hooked me up with the organisers of a closed Facebook group for Australians with chronic myeloid leukaemia. I'd never really grasped the appeal of Facebook. I rarely checked it, as over the years I'd somehow managed to become 'friends' with scores of people I'd never met. I'd get random notifications alerting me that my year four classmate had changed her status from 'single' to 'in a relationship', or someone I chatted to at a hotel pool in Bali back in 2007 was celebrating their birthday in two days.

I've always lived by the philosophy that if a person wouldn't think to visit you in hospital if you were sick, then they probably weren't a close friend. And let's face it, not everyone has to be a best friend. Acquaintances are great, but the days when people came in and out of your life at the right time are long gone.

Now they're forever connected to you; an echo on your social media feed. You might not care what your ex-boyfriend's sister is up to anymore, but you still know how she takes her coffee, her dog's name, and who she thinks deserves to win the latest season of *Survivor*.

So I was reticent to join, thinking I'd be hit with a fresh wave of inane notifications alerting me to viral videos of stupid people doing stupid things, and uninformed online arguments about the Syrian civil war.

But it turned out to be a lifeline. Up until my diagnosis I'd never even heard of chronic myeloid leukaemia. I'd never met anyone with it, or spoken to anybody knowledgeable about it. So having a group of regular people to share my questions, fears and updates with was a huge comfort. At the time of writing this I have only ever met one person with CML, but I feel as though I'm part of a close-knit group who I can trust and confide in when I'm at my lowest, when I'm scared, confused and when I just want to vent.

It was through these forums that I connected with Sharyn, a single mother of two who had been diagnosed with CML six years prior. Sharyn was one of the unlucky ones whose cancer didn't respond to the TKI drugs which had saved so many lives in the fifteen years since their introduction. She was involved in a trial with Professor Hughes, which required her to relocate to Adelaide to undergo treatment. Despite the uncertainty which hung over her like a black cloud, the pretty blonde's positivity never waned, and in the first few months after my diagnosis she became a great support, advising me on everything from what foods and skincare products to use to treat medication side effects, and how my life would change as a result of this illness.

She also seemed to know exactly the right time to drop me a private message to check in and see how I was doing.

'Been thinking about you lately—are you coping ok?' she would write. It was these brief notes which often turned around a bad day into a not-so-bad day, and I'll be forever grateful.

Another of my CML Facebook friends was, in fact, the mother of a teenage boy with CML. I couldn't imagine how hard it would be for a parent to be dealt a blow like that. The helplessness would be unbearable. Fortunately, this particular form of leukaemia is more an older person's disease, but I was still surprised at how many young women were part of this online group, many of them struggling with issues around starting families.

Some had managed to have children in the years following their diagnosis, having stopped taking their medication for a while in order to conceive. For some, who had reached the stage of complete molecular remission (a target every CML patient hopes to achieve), their cancer continued to lay dormant even after they had given birth, and they could stay off the medication indefinitely. Others weren't so lucky and had to recommence their treatment as soon as their baby was born.

Posts would often cover topics of side effects, with members asking the group if they believed a certain side effect was CML or medication related or otherwise, and whether anyone else had experienced it since their diagnosis. Most members of the group had moved beyond vanity and had no qualms about posting photos of themselves sporting puffy eyes, gross skin rashes, bald patches on heads and open wounds. It was such an honest way to compare notes and get the group's opinion as to whether said problem required a trip to the emergency department or just a bit of antiseptic cream.

I joined three Facebook groups a few months after that fateful week, one just for women with CML, one for Aussies, and an international group.

Hearing about the experiences of people in other countries made me feel so grateful to live in Australia. Sure, we complain about the state of our healthcare system, and it could always do with more funding for hospital upgrades, wages and emergency services, but we are so fortunate. In the United States, tyrosine kinase inhibitors—the drugs used to treat CML—can cost leukaemia patients thousands of dollars a month. In 2015, it was reported in newspapers and medical journals by a group of British researchers that a year's supply of Gleevec (generic name imatinib mesylate) cost just US$159 to produce, but was being sold for US$106,322.

But thanks to Australia's Pharmaceutical Benefits Scheme, nilotinib—the tyrosine kinase inhibitor I would eventually take to prolong my life—would cost me less than $50 a month. I often joke to Nick that it'd be a good idea to start stockpiling them in case of a global catastrophe, because I wouldn't last long without them. The cancer would simply relaunch its assault on my body and I'd eventually waste away and die. Unless, like in the film *World War Z*, a virus turned the population into flesh-eating zombies. In the movie, Brad Pitt's character injects himself with a deadly virus after learning the zombies only attacked healthy people, in order to make himself 'invisible' to them and save the world.

'I'd be invincible!' I said to Nick after we watched the action flick.

'Well, not really,' I added, 'but at least I wouldn't be turned into the walking dead. *You'd* be in trouble though!'

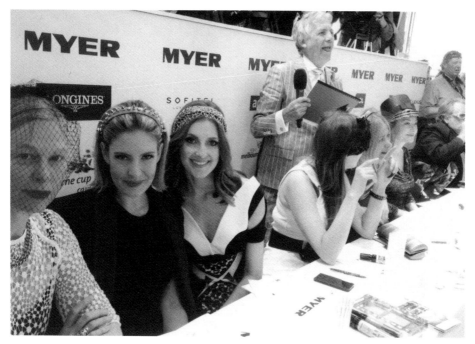

Judging Myer Fashions on the Field alongside designer Kate Sylvester and Kate Waterhouse at Flemington's Melbourne Cup Day in 2013.

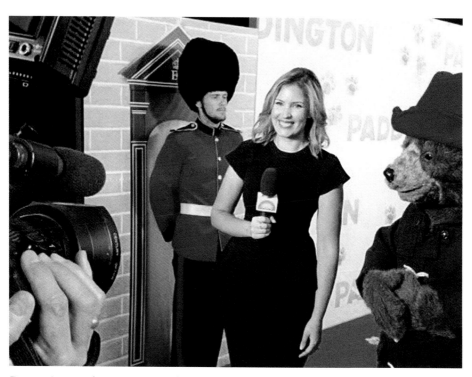

Reporting at the premiere of *Paddington* for Nine's *Weekend Today* in 2014.

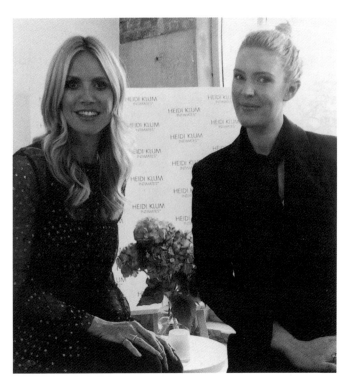

Interviewing German Supermodel Heidi Klum about her latest range of intimates in 2016.

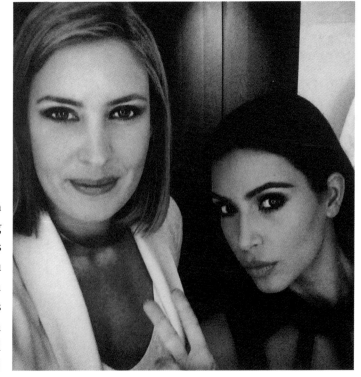

Kim Kardashian and I taking bathroom selfies together. As you can see from the photo, she's clearly much more practised at it than me!

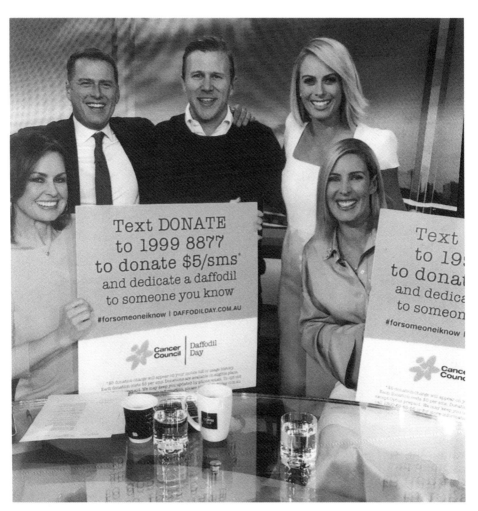

Appearing on Channel Nine's *Today* show for Daffodil Day 2016, the day my story was published in *The Daily Telegraph*. I was so overcome with emotion I can't even remember this photo being taken.

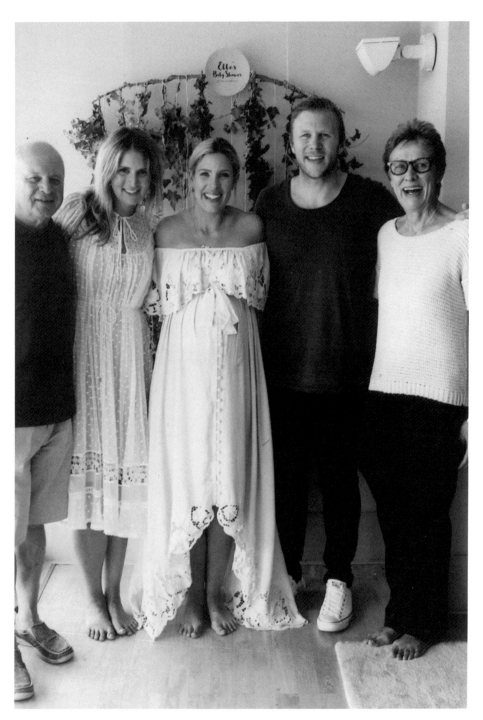

Celebrating my baby shower with Nick and my in-laws. Nick's dad Peter (far left), my sister-in-law Chrissy Collingwood Boots (second from left), Nick, and Nick's mum Hettie (far right). Chrissy, who is an event-planning genius, put on the most incredible party for me. I felt like a celebrity!

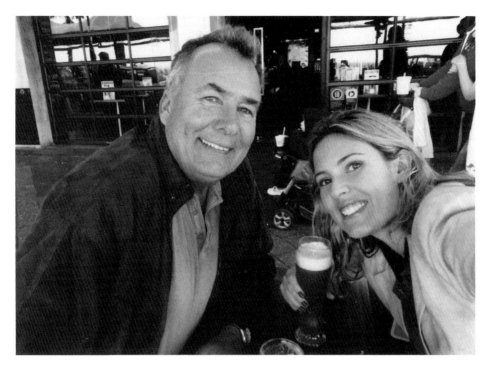

This pic was taken a few years after Dad was diagnosed with prostate cancer.

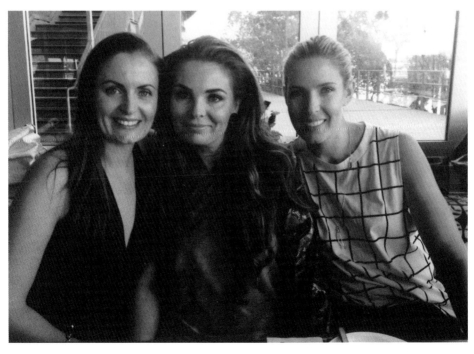

Me with my beautiful sisters Amy (far left) and Martine (centre).

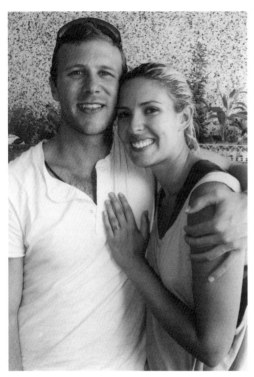

Nick proposed to me a few hours before this pic was taken of us on Christmas Eve 2011. We sent this photo to our family and friends.

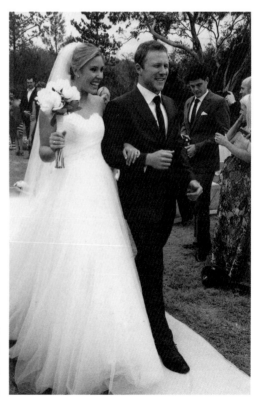

Our wedding day in November 2012. The weather held off and I still remember it as one of the best days of my life.

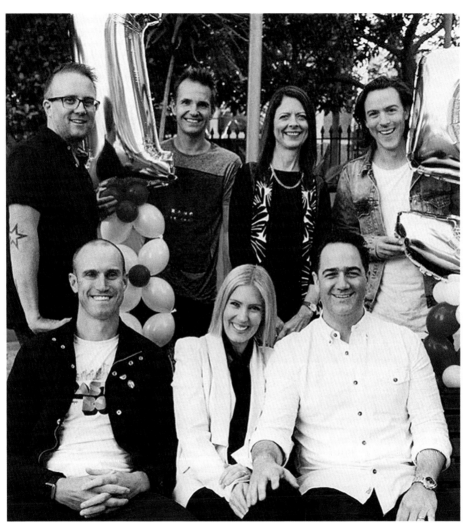

Celebrating Nova Entertainment's 15-year anniversary in March 2016: with my Nova colleagues. Clockwise from left: Jonathon J.Mo Moran, Kent Smallzy Small, Nova CEO Cathy O'Connor, Tim Blackwell, Michael Wippa Wipfli, me and Ryan Fitzy Fitzgerald.

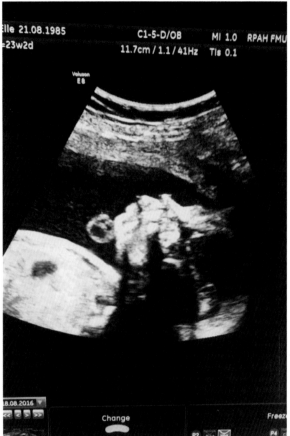

Tor's 23-week ultrasound. Seeing his cute button nose so clearly for the first time was so incredible.

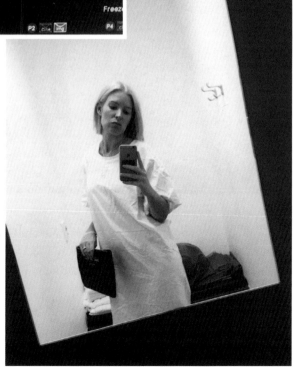

Trying to make light of an awful situation. Taking a selfie in the Royal Prince Alfred Hospital's changing room ahead of my bone marrow biopsy.

The Detox

'Where are the frying pans?' Nick asked me a few days after our appointment with Professor Hughes. He'd just returned from a run and was holding a bowl of scrambled eggs as he searched the kitchen cupboards for something to cook them in.

'They were Teflon, so I've sold them,' I said casually, pointing to a cardboard box sitting at the front door. 'Someone bought them from Gumtree for $80; they're picking them up tonight. I sold all our pots too. We do have a stainless steel one left if you need one for your breakfast—it's in the second drawer down.'

Beside the pots and pans was another open box, filled with an assortment of half-empty bottles of cleaning sprays, fabric softeners and other cleaning aids. I'd also filled a reusable plastic shopping bag to the brim with plastic containers and kitchen utensils, which sat amongst the kitchen detritus.

Nick surveyed the neatly arranged midden, and raised his eyebrows. He walked back into the kitchen and began methodically opening and closing all the drawers and cupboards.

'What are you doing with all our bloody stuff?' he finally asked.

A trickle of paranoia had begun to meander through my mind in the days immediately after my diagnosis. The Prof had assured me my illness had not been caused by my lifestyle, and was simply an unfortunate cellular fuck-up—but it didn't stop me questioning my past and present choices, and wondering if there was something I'd done that had triggered my sickness.

I had always been pretty healthy. I was a moderate drinker, enjoying a glass or two of red wine during the week and a few more on a weekend. I reserved junk food for rare Sunday morning hangovers and parties, but during the week my diet consisted of yoghurt and berries for breakfast, a chicken and avocado salad or sandwich for lunch and a couple of coffees throughout the day. Dinners could be anything from marinated chicken with steamed vegetables to sashimi, salads and slow-cooked beef stew.

But when it came to cosmetics and household cleaning, I rarely checked the packaging for ingredients and blindly used whatever smelled the nicest or was the most effective at making me and my home look nice.

About once a year I would eagerly sign up to a new fitness regimen like F45, CrossFit or Barre, only to revert back after a few months to walking and the odd yoga class, having reminded myself that I did, in fact, hate exercising for the sake of exercise. I recently came across an Instagram post which perfectly described my body type: *Not terrible, but definitely enjoys pasta.*

My diet and lifestyle had greatly improved with age. As a child and teenager, I ate terribly. Mum cooked healthy dinners, but white bread and Coca-Cola was readily available at home, and I had a severe addiction to gummy bears. By the age of ten I already had gained a mouthful of fillings courtesy of my very, very sweet tooth.

I hated drinking water, and for the three years I attended Pymble Ladies' College in my early teens, my breakfast consisted of a can of V energy drink and a bacon and cheese roll from the Pymble railway station bakery. I shudder to think what that did to my developing body.

Sport was also something that didn't come naturally to me. Nobody in my family was particularly sporty, and while I always tried my best at school sports I was rarely picked for the team.

I gave netball, softball and even cricket a try, hoping to find some kind of activity I wasn't completely uncoordinated at. I readily signed up to Saturday sport with my girlfriends, but never made the same teams as them. At netball try-outs, almost all of my friends would be picked for the A-grade team, while I'd be lucky to be chosen for C or D grade. The only year they had enough teams to warrant an E grade, I joined that one too.

One year I did get to join my friends, playing softball. Our team was called the Pittwater Dolphins and, unsurprisingly, I was almost always sent into the outfield. I lasted one season.

Swimming was the only thing I was remotely good at. As a kid I would spend hours in the pool, and in year five even made it to the regional swimming finals for backstroke, where I finished second last. My moderate skill in the pool convinced me I would also be good at Nippers. I enrolled at Newport Surf Life Saving Club, and each Sunday would join my girlfriend Kristy on the sand, where we would line up in our group, plonk on our yellow and maroon striped patrol caps and do a bunch of activities. I sucked at 'Flags', which involved racing along the beach and grabbing a hard piece of hose. There would be one hose fewer than the number of Nippers competing, and I usually came up empty handed.

I stuck at it, until the end of the second summer. It was one of the last days of the season, and the weather was miserable. A storm had come through the night before, causing a swell with six-foot waves, which, to a twelve-year-old, looked more like mini tsunamis. Our instructor pointed to a foam buoy about 80 metres out to sea, and informed us we had to paddle around it and head back into shore. I tried to think of a reason why I couldn't compete, but I was so petrified my brain had stopped functioning.

My girlfriend Kristy didn't seem too worried, and I desperately didn't want to look like a chicken in front of the group, so I took a deep breath, picked up my foam board and dived into the surf. By some miracle I managed to make it past the towering surf break and reach the buoy. *I've totally got this*, I told myself as I cruised around the marker. I was one of the last in the water, but I wasn't *dead* last for a change. I paddled towards the shore and turned back to the horizon, hoping to find a small wave to ride back in on. All of a sudden my board was picked up by a huge swell and was thrust towards the beach—but only for a moment. The wave broke and my board nosedived straight into the shallow water. I tumbled through the surf, swallowing a mix of salty liquid and sand, thinking I'd never surface: I was going to die! As I dragged myself up onto the shore, too exhausted to bother walking to the finish line, I vowed to give up any pretension of sportiness. It was too dangerous.

'I hope our kids get your temperament,' Nick would often say to me, 'but I really don't want them to inherit your athleticism.'

I knew I couldn't make amends for my past dietary indiscretions and poor fitness, but I could ensure that my child, if he or she miraculously survived, would have the healthiest start possible. And hopefully have a little more interest in getting its heart rate up than its mum.

◆ ◆ ◆

Fortunately, the first few months of 2016 had put me in good stead for this somewhat premature pregnancy. I had already begun reading Lana and David Asprey's *The Better Baby Book*, and had adjusted my eating habits to prepare my body for baby-growing. Slow-cooked bone broth soups, oily fish, and steamed vegetables loaded with organic grass-fed butter were now regular dinner options, while breakfast featured biodynamic eggs or plain Greek yoghurt, berries and homemade granola.

But whereas before 1 April I wouldn't have thought twice about hoeing into the occasional promotional cupcake or treat sent to the office by a savvy publicist, I was now terrified of unknown foodstuffs. Artificial flavours, preservatives, sugar substitutes and hydrogenated fats became the enemy, and I developed an aversion to eating out. I would fret over the cooking methods, wondering if any ingredients had been microwaved in a plastic container or fried in a non-stick pan. I stopped short of asking to check out the kitchen, but it did cross my mind once or twice.

Takeaway was out of the question, as I couldn't bear the idea of hot food coming into contact with cheap plastic containers, which I was sure contained bisphenol A (BPA) or bisphenol S (BPS), compounds which some studies have suggested can mimic oestrogen in the body and cause breast cancer cells to multiply.

My chemophobia also extended to skincare and cosmetics. I had amassed an impressive cosmetics cupboard during my years covering fashion and beauty, and spent a whole afternoon sorting through dozens of skincare creams and mascaras, putting anything unused into a bag which I donated to a charity called The Beauty Bank. Anything containing parabens, sodium laureth sulfate, triclosan or synthetic fragrances were binned, leaving surprisingly few items with which to beautify myself.

I switched to fluoride-free toothpaste, swapped my anti-perspirant for natural deodorant paste, and ditched my moisturiser in favour of extra virgin coconut and rosehip oils. My lip balm was beeswax-based, and I had swapped my beloved MAC Studio Fix foundation for an organic-based alternative.

After a few days, I had officially completed my transformation from *Toxic Thirty-Something* to *Crazy, Hippy and Pregnant Cancer Lady*.

Nick was surprisingly ok with my household overhaul. Occasionally I'd come home to the distinct smell of chlorine bleach, Nick having found a stray cleaning product with which to substitute my probiotic toilet cleaner. I couldn't chastise him for doing a bit of cleaning, so I kept my mouth shut, but usually managed to track down the offending product and discreetly chuck it in the bin.

I knew I was teetering on the verge of developing full-blown orthorexia, which was far from a healthy psychological state. But having things like trans fats and sulphites to worry about had proved an effective distraction from the bigger problems I was facing.

◆ ◆ ◆

'Mum, these are way too expensive!' I said as we stood together in front of a collection of All-Clad pots and pans at Victoria's Basement.

'I said I wanted to buy them for you, honey. Please let me,' she pleaded. 'I feel so helpless, and I know this is something you really need.'

Mum had flown down to Sydney a couple of days after my diagnosis, and Nick's parents had offered to have her stay upstairs with them for as long as she wanted.

It had been such a blessing having Het and Pete so close. Every night that first week Het had cooked for us. She'd done our washing, cleaned the apartment and fed the cat when I just couldn't muster the energy. I already knew I'd scored in the mother-in-law department, but this was truly beyond the call of duty and I was so grateful.

Mum had already begun looking for a unit to rent in Sydney's inner west. I had no idea what the next few months would bring, but Mum would feel better knowing she was close by in case I needed her.

She'd been nagging me to give her things to do to assist me, but with Het organising the domestic side of things, there wasn't much more Mum *could* do, so she wanted to contribute financially.

The shopping trip had been a welcome distraction for us both. I knew Mum was struggling to keep her emotions in check. I'd made a concerted effort to remain positive in front of my family. It was self-preservation: I was balancing on an emotional tightrope of the finest wire, and knew it would take just a single tear from a loved one to tip me back into a pit of desolation. If I seemed optimistic, none of my loved ones felt they had the right to be miserable in front of me, I surmised. It had formed a delicate circle, which Mum broke that afternoon.

She lost it in the car, after we'd inspected a unit in Lilyfield. The place had felt cold and unwelcoming—unlike Mum's quaint weatherboard home in Brisbane, which she had over the years transformed into a cosy sanctuary, smelling of English breakfast tea and gardenias.

'I didn't like the vibe in that place,' I said, closing the front door of the rundown unit block behind me. We got to her car, a 12-year-old black Holden Astra, which she refused to trade in despite its dodgy motor. I slipped into the passenger's seat, and I turned to her. 'You know, you don't need to stay in Sydney,' I said. 'Het is here if I need help with anything. You're only an hour's flight away, and it's ridiculous for you to be paying rent if you're not prepared to have someone move into your place to help with the cost. Realistically, you can't afford it . . .'

'Mum?' I prompted, after she didn't respond. She hadn't started the car up, and was sitting beside me silently. I looked over and could see her shoulders shaking.

'Oh Mum, it's ok,' I said, reaching over to hug her.

She couldn't hold the tears back anymore, and they began to pour from her eyes. I hated seeing her upset; it crushed me.

'I feel so helpless!' she managed between shuddering sobs. 'I just want to take it away from you! You're too young to have to go through this.'

She'd been so strong since she had arrived, offering encouraging words whenever I relayed details of our visit to the Prof or found out more about my leukaemia.

I knew she was struggling; that she had cried herself to sleep, like me, when nobody was around. My diagnosis had dredged up the same emotions she had battled after the death of my brother, Eric, forty years ago. The idea of another child dying would have been unbearable.

I felt a tear fall from my eye. I wiped it away, but another replaced it and soon they were falling freely down my face.

'I'm so sorry, Elle,' Mum said when she saw my jaw shiver as I tried to suppress my grief. 'It's going to be fine, and if you would prefer me to stay in Brisbane then I will. I just want you to know I'm here, and I love you so, so much.'

We sat, holding each other outside the blond-brick unit block until our fragile smiles returned. I turned the Holden Astra's CD player on, and flicked to Queen's 'A Kind Of Magic', one of our favourite songs.

'I'll be alright, Mum,' I said, turning up the volume on the upbeat track. 'I come from tough stock.'

◆ ◆ ◆

I sat down with Rhett Watson, the paper's managing editor, to discuss my options. I knew I couldn't go back to working 10–12-hour days. I needed to shift my priorities and put my health, and my pregnancy, at the top of the list, and prepare my mind for the fight that lay ahead.

Perhaps it was because I was now aware of what was happening inside me, but in the weeks post-diagnosis I began to notice a growing weariness in my body, an exhaustion that no amount of sleep could shake. I became, for the first time in my life, a napper. If I didn't rest each afternoon I would crash into bed about 6 p.m. and sleep through until the next morning.

I hadn't picked up a paintbrush since the week I was diagnosed. I was usually too tired to do much at the end of each day anyway, but I'd developed a fear of my paints. I'd been spending hours inhaling noxious-smelling oil paints and the equally fumey turpentine cleaning agent in the lead-up to my diagnosis, and I couldn't help thinking it had played a part in causing my cancer. The idea that something I loved so much could have harmed me was quite devastating, and had put me off even sketching with lead pencils.

I'll be forever grateful to Rhett, Mick and Dorey—my bosses at News Corp—for the support they gave me in those first months. I felt so much guilt at not being able to work at my previous pace, but they allowed me to take the time I needed for rest and medical appointments. I arranged with Rhett that I would work for three days at home, and two in the office. It was approaching winter, and spending hours on crammed buses and amongst snuffling colleagues was the last thing I needed to deal with in light of my compromised health.

My new commute-free workdays freed up my time, allowing me to take a long walk in the morning and then rest in the afternoon. I would continue to file my double-page fashion column, Code Red celebrity fashion page and Saturday features each week, and contribute fashion news to Sydney Confidential if I was able.

◆ ◆ ◆

What began as fifteen-minute strolls around the block soon turned into eight-kilometre hikes. Being outdoors made my world seem bigger, my life more inconsequential as I counted the hundreds of people driving to work, oblivious to my predicament and distracted by their own struggles, desires and dreams.

Being outdoors also made me feel more alive. Every time I stepped out our front door and felt the chill of the dewy winter air, I was reminded how lucky I was to be upright, limber and alive. I wasn't horizontal on an uncomfortable hospital bed, perforated by needles and tubes—at least not right now. Today I was ok. Tomorrow could be different, but today I had goosebumps from the morning breeze. Today I could feel the dew of the morning grass tickling my ankles as I wandered around my front garden.

It's said that pregnancy heightens the senses, so perhaps that's why life suddenly seemed more vivid. The world was in high definition. I'd switched over from analogue to digital, and it felt kind of amazing.

My feet often took me to Callan Park—an expansive, leafy haven on the banks of the Parramatta River beside Canada Bay's popular Bay Run walking track.

I'd discovered a number of beautiful areas around my relatively new neighbourhood since I had begun my walks, and the former hospital for the insane was undoubtedly my favourite place to wander and ponder.

It was easy to spend hours meandering among the old sandstone and dilapidated weatherboard buildings on the 61-hectare grounds, each walk uncovering a new refuge to sit and meditate. The eeriness of the broken, weary buildings, and the deep shadowed groves of ancient Moreton Bay figs and jacarandas made Callan Park not a welcoming place after dark, but there was an undeniable romance to the place at 7 a.m. on a misty morning, which was my favourite time to visit.

Each morning I'd rug up in a beanie, thick leggings and a long-sleeved top. I'd finish with an oversized black hoodie, stuffing its pockets with my iPhone, headphones, a few dollars and a house key. I'd drink two large glasses of chilled water before I left, my thoughts fixed on the decaf coffee and green juice I would reward myself with once my phone's health app alerted me that I had reached 4000 steps.

I had spent the first few weeks of my daily walks trying to forget about my situation. I ignored the twinges in my belly and tried to focus on the beats and lyrics emanating from my ear buds as they played the latest hits from Selena Gomez and One Direction. Trying to determine what feelings Justin Timberlake just couldn't stop or which ex-boyfriend Taylor Swift was singing about proved better distractions than the devastatingly beautiful but equally depressing lyrics of Angus & Julia Stone.

It soon became difficult to ignore the fact I wasn't alone on my walks. I'd catch myself unconsciously touching my stomach as I wandered through the back streets of Drummoyne and Balmain, wondering who this unseen walking partner was, or would be.

I pictured my hands grasping a pram and pushing it along this same route, wondering if the blueberry-sized embryo would enjoy this ritual if it ever made it out of its watery, dark world.

I began humming along to my pop playlist, hoping to share whatever song was playing with my walking buddy as we traipsed along the Iron Cove Bridge and watched the ferries shuttle white-collar workers and tourists towards the city.

My walks often involved wandering the streets of Rozelle, and on Saturdays I would head to the markets at Rozelle Public School, taking my time browsing the stalls selling antique knick-knacks, collectable books, handmade furniture and vintage jewellery.

One Saturday in June, I stopped by a large stall selling an assortment of crystals and gems. On one side, a shelving unit sagged under the weight of dozens of rockmelon-sized egg geodes which had been split in half to expose their magical, crystallised innards. The centre of the stall was laden with small, compartmentalised trays filled with variously sized stones of tiger's eye, rose and clear quartz, tourmaline, lapis lazuli and jade, each tray's compartment sporting a faded, hand-written description of each stone and the ailments and disorders they were believed to treat.

'Excuse me, I was wondering if you have any stones for blood issues?' I asked the stall owner.

'Hi there. Yeah that'd be the blood stone you'd be after, darl,' he replied. The man, in his late sixties, seemed distracted by something going on over my shoulder. 'Sorry, love,' he said, his eyes continuing to scan over my shoulder. 'One of our regulars has turned up and he's got a bit of a habit of leaving with a few souvenirs if ya know what I mean,' he said, giving me a knowing wink.

'Take your time,' I said, giving a gentle laugh, then asked if he could find me a blood stone pendant or bracelet—something I could wear.

'I've got an African blood stone for ya, love. Good for anaemia and the like,' he said, untangling a few leather necklaces from a tall stand laden with colourful gemstones, and handing me a deep green stone pendant with red flecks.

'I'll take it, thanks,' I said, putting the string over my head. The small, hexagonal stone felt cold against my bare decolletage, but quickly warmed up as it absorbed my body heat.

◆ ◆ ◆

I've always had a healthy scepticism for alternative therapies, but never closed myself off to different methods of healing.

Numerous studies have proven the benefits of acupuncture and meditation, and when you've got cancer or a chronic illness, there's little you won't consider if there's a chance it could make some kind of positive difference to your health.

A few months prior to my diagnosis, I'd arranged a naturo-pathic consultation at a detox clinic in Bondi, to get some advice on the vitamins I should be taking for my fertility. The centre offered a range of new-age treatments such as colonic hydro-therapy and 3D body imaging. I met with the naturopath, a pleasantly spoken, petite blonde woman in her early forties.

'To get a better idea of what's going on, I'm going to start by using this new machine which scans your body at a cellular level,' she explained. 'It's called a Mini Quantum Magnetic Resonance Analyzer. We sent staff over to Germany to get trained in how to use it; it really is an amazing technology.'

I immediately thought of the Ashton Kutcher film, *Dude, Where's My Car?*, in which a bunch of aliens are sent to Earth to retrieve a device called the Continuum Transfunctioner. I hoped that despite its stupid name, the Mini Quantum

Magnetic Resonance Analyzer was a little more scientifically sound.

She asked me to remove all my jewellery, then handed me a thick metal probe the same size and shape as a tennis racquet handle. 'Hold it until it beeps, and then we'll check the results,' she said, turning on a small machine connected to the device. She brought up a web page on her computer which showed a human figure and a bunch of graphs.

My bullshit radar had popped up the moment my fingers had clasped around the metal probe, but I was curious to see how it played out.

The machine determined that I was having troubles with my gall bladder and right wrist, and I needed to eat fewer soy products. My wrist felt fine, as did my gall bladder, but I'll admit I did love me some soy sauce.

Funnily enough, blood cancer or bone issues didn't make an appearance on my list of ailments, even though my body would have been in the throes of a bone-marrow meltdown at the time. The naturopath gave me a printout of the results, prescribed me a list of pricey vitamins, and $330 later suggested I come back in a few weeks for a follow-up.

I really wanted to give her the benefit of the doubt, but decided to do some digging into this quantum machine—a very easy task, thanks to the website address at the bottom of the printout I'd received, which quickly confirmed my suspicions.

'Mini quantum magnetic resonance analyzer is one of the latest and most persuasive sales tools; in the marketing process,' a blurb on the site read. 'Just 1 minute, sub-health testing services, the accuracy of the instrument to allow customers to be immediately convinced, and conducive to sales staff to communicate further with the customer, so that guests are willing to accept your products is the best tool for sales and wealth doubled.'

If the poor grammar didn't scream SCAM, the words themselves certainly did. I emailed the supplier for a quote to buy one of the machines, and discovered the products came from China, not Germany—and to obtain one of these high-tech health devices I simply had to hand over US$250.

I thought about asking the naturopath for a refund, but laughed it off as an expensive lesson. I had other stuff to get on with.

Post-diagnosis me would have had a very different reaction. A well-meaning friend contacted me on Facebook when she found out about my illness. She told me about a machine called a Spooky2 Rife which promised to heal the body by using 'quantum entanglement to affect DNA'. I watched a video about it on my way into work, and for a fleeting moment almost managed to convince myself that perhaps it wouldn't be completely ridiculous to spend $700 on this 'miracle machine'.

After my diagnosis, I quickly realised that people with cancer—particularly terminal or incurable, chronic cancers like mine—can be extremely vulnerable. When we are at our lowest it can be so tempting to believe a superfood or a seemingly magical energy device could be the miracle cure we've been waiting for the medical community to discover. But while some people truly believe their snake-oil potions offer the cure-all to disease, there are probably just as many who are simply opportunists looking to cash in on people's fear and desperation.

The uncertainty of what would take place in the months following my pregnancy news had caused me to defer my studies into nutrition, but I vowed to myself that if I ever did completely delve into nutrition and wellness coaching, I'd steer clear of fancy sounding contraptions and 'miracle treatments'.

I had no delusions my African bloodstone necklace would cure my cancer, but it became a talisman of sorts, and I became superstitious about it, wearing it at all times.

◆ ◆ ◆

Fortunately the nausea I was anticipating as I progressed through the first trimester was tolerable and intermittent. I didn't have any strange pregnancy cravings, save for the occasional desire for oranges, bread and tasty cheese (fortunately not together). Early on I'd been living on stewed meat, salads, eggs and fresh juices, but one morning, when I was about eight weeks pregnant, I woke up feeling as though I'd go crazy if I didn't get my teeth around a chewy piece of cheddar-topped sourdough. So I drove to an organic supermarket in Rozelle, and the moment I returned to the car park I slid into the front seat of the car, tore the bread stick in half, broke off a chunk of organic cheese with my hands and proceeded to demolish both, too ravenous to wait until I could eat them politely at a table, covering myself in a light dusting of flour and cheese crumbs. It gave me the hiccups, but the satisfaction I felt from that in-car meal was like nothing I'd experienced before.

In those early weeks, I didn't suffer too many adverse effects as a result of the pregnancy, or the cancer, but I did notice one positive side effect, one night in bed. I'd slipped between the sheets and noticed how my body felt instantly ready for sleep.

It wasn't whirring with thoughts of how much I needed to get done and how little time I had to do it, or thinking about what stupid things I'd said or done that day, or would probably say or do the following one. My heart wasn't thumping erratically and my lungs felt clear, strong and cavernous.

My anxiety had disappeared.

I realised I hadn't felt that awful suffocating sensation in weeks. I'd been too busy focusing on my life, and the new life inside me, to concern myself with thoughts about not having emptied the dishwasher, or having failed to order more cat litter. Whenever such thoughts had surfaced, I automatically said to myself: *You have leukaemia, Elle. What's the worst thing that can happen if you don't get this unimportant but urgent thing done? Is anyone going to die? Are you going to care about this in a year's time, or even a week's time?*

The dozens of self-help books I'd consumed over the years, the neuro-linguistic programming guides on positive self-talk I'd studied, and the advice from counsellors and psychologists had automatically clicked into gear the moment I was diagnosed.

I was finally able to breathe, and think clearly and rationally, without the worry and anxiousness I'd lived with for a decade.

That realisation was a life-changing moment for me.

I marvelled at how experiencing a trauma could have such a positive effect on a person's mental health. It seemed so counterintuitive, and yet it was so very true for me.

I was curious to know whether I was just an odd case, or whether it was a common response to a traumatic event. I reached out to Avanti Singh, a psychologist in Sydney who also specialises in Ayurveda and meditation.

Ms Singh was far from shocked when I told her of what I considered my somewhat miraculous mental health recovery.

'I'm not surprised by that at all,' she said. 'We become unhealthy and we become unwell when there's disconnection to the body. The body is present and thoughts are in two places: the past or in the future. That's what yogic teaching and traditions espouse.'

The registered psychologist explained that traumatic events—particularly those involving an illness or health crisis—can often bring the mind back to the present moment.

It made so much sense. I couldn't foresee what my future held, and I had no way of knowing what could have triggered my cancer, so I was forced just to take my illness and pregnancy moment by moment.

I had been practising mindfulness without even realising it.

The Let Down

Why me? It's a question almost everybody who has been dealt a blow inevitably asks themselves.

For some, the question is more an accusation, a curse at the universe or whatever higher power they believe in for dealing them such an unfair hand.

But as the dust storm of my situation started to settle in my mind, I began to pose this question out of genuine curiosity. Why, out of the billions of people on earth, did *I* get this rare illness?

According to the American Cancer Society, there were just four risk factors associated with chronic myeloid leukaemia:

being male; being older; having lived near the site of an atomic bomb blast or nuclear reactor incident; and having undergone prior chemotherapy treatment.

I felt cheated. Not one single risk factor applied to me.

In 2015 *The Daily Telegraph* had run a story about cancer statistics, which had for some reason caught my eye. It said a US study had concluded that about two-thirds of cancers were caused by random mutations, rather than external environmental factors. For most of us, it surmised, getting cancer was just bad luck.

I had conflicting feelings about the study's conclusion. I'd heard stories of the most disciplined health junkies being diagnosed with brain tumours, while heavy smokers and drinkers reached triple-digit birthdays. Case in point was my Granny, who at 92 could have run rings around most 70-year-olds despite living off a diet of dry sherry, Horizon 40s and the odd sandwich. Would this encourage people to throw their diets and exercise regimens out the window, knowing that however cleanly they lived their lives there was a chance they'd get cancer anyway? Or would they be more vigilant about living a clean lifestyle, knowing they had given themselves the best chance of preventing cancer, even if it eventually did come knocking?

I may have just been unlucky, but deep down I knew there was one risk factor the studies hadn't factored in: stress.

On the scale of stressful jobs, writing entertainment and fashion at *The Telegraph* might not have shared top billing with roles like Prime Minister or neurosurgeon, but it was intense. Daily deadlines, the pressure to ensure every detail was correct before a million or more people read it, and the worry that at any moment your position could be ripped from under you certainly kept the cortisol running.

My predisposition to panic added another layer to the mix, creating a potent cocktail of nervousness I found difficult to deal with at times. I could hide it, superficially suppress it, but the adrenaline still rushed under the surface no matter how calm and collected I tried to appear to my peers and bosses.

Waking up in the middle of the night, wondering if I had triple-checked names, dates and details was a common occurrence. I'd lie there running the story through my mind, wondering if it was too late to call the news desk and make changes before the final edition went to the printers.

Most of the time, I'd arrive at work to find there was no mistake, and the three hours of lost sleep had all been for nothing.

I knew most of my stress was self-inflicted. I'd worry what my bosses thought of my work that week—whether I'd done enough to garner their favour, or if they were plotting to replace me on account of my recent lack of page-three story options.

My adrenals were firing constantly during my work week, only to inevitably crash and burn the moment I switched off, throwing my immune system into chaos.

I can't remember being well during a vacation or work break in the past seven years. Every time I went on leave, I would fall ill with some kind of bug. My situation was not at all uncommon. In fact, there's a name for it: the 'let down effect'. Studies have found that many people experience more flare-ups in illness and pain *after*, as opposed to *during*, stressful periods. It's believed the hormones responsible for suppressing pain and firing up the immune system are activated during times of acute stress. This would have given our ancestors an advantage when it came to fleeing danger or attacking predators—but humans weren't designed to remain in this 'fight or flight' mode for long. The inflammatory effect of cortisol and various hormones on the body has been well documented, and linked to a raft of illnesses such as arthritis and multiple sclerosis.

'The fight–flight–freeze response can create all sorts of havoc within the body: increased heart rate, increased blood pressure, stress hormone release, rapid breathing and weakened immunity,' Sydney psychologist Avanti Singh explains. 'All disease is caused by inflammation; I think most medical practitioners would agree with this.'

Looking back at the months leading up to my diagnosis, there were definitely signs that something wasn't right. The telltale symptoms of leukaemia—the bruising, bone pain and enlarged spleen—were absent, but there were plenty of other alarm bells. Just before my thirtieth birthday, I managed to convince myself I had a neurological disease.

'My hands are malfunctioning,' I told a young GP in Bondi, as I sat on the edge of his white examination bed, legs dangling. I usually went to see Doc, but didn't have my car that day, and was desperate to speak to someone about it.

I held up my hands, palms facing the floor, and watched as they trembled. I explained that I'd begun feeling a tingling and numbness in my fingers and the side of my face. 'It kind of feels like they're not my hands,' I explained, looking at them quizzically. 'Like they're not attached properly anymore. I'm pretty sure I've got multiple sclerosis or something.'

I'm sure I wasn't his first patient to self-diagnose with a serious disease courtesy of Google, but he gave a good poker face.

He asked me to do a bunch of strange exercises: poking my tongue out, making 'jazz hands', and following his finger around with only my eyes. With his short blond hair and Bondi tan, the young doctor looked like he should be *playing* one on a TV soap. His good looks made me feel a bit self-conscious as I waved my hands around like someone competing in a rock eisteddfod.

'Look, I don't think you've got anything serious neurologically,' he said, finally.

'If we book you in for an MRI, the problem is everyone's brains are slightly different. We could find some anomaly that actually isn't a problem, but looks like it could be. It could open up a can of worms, and you definitely don't want that. I suggest you wait a few weeks and see if the sensations disappear. If they get worse, come back and we can take another look.'

I felt better knowing there was nothing obviously wrong going on in my brain, but the strange feelings didn't disappear.

The worry had started to affect my sleep, and my work, and the intense shortness of breath had also returned with a vengeance, making it hard to concentrate. I'd accrued almost two months of annual leave, so I decided to book myself into a health retreat.

I did some research and settled on a quaint retreat in the town of Bundanoon called Solar Springs, two hours by train from Sydney. The last thing I wanted was to run into a celebrity trying to 'find herself' with vegan soups and savasanas and feeling obliged to hit her up for an interview in the meditation room. If the editor discovered I'd been practising my downward dogs beside Miley Cyrus and hadn't at least taken a few sneaky shots on my iPhone, I may as well have handed in my resignation on the spot.

Solar Springs offered the holy retreat trinity—limited phone service, a cosy spot to read, and a remedial massage or two. And it was affordable. It was just what I was looking for.

As soon as the train had left the graffiti-decorated walls of Sydney's Central Station and began its journey along the Southern Highlands line, I felt the nervous tension start to slip away, and by the time I stepped onto the tiny, heritage railway platform at Bundanoon my shoulders had dropped below my jaw line for what felt like the first time in months.

At the retreat I dumped my bags on the double bed in the small, spartan room I'd be staying in for the next five days. 'You'll be able to see the kangaroos from here in the late afternoon,' a staff member named Sue explained, pointing to a small window in my room which overlooked a lush valley and a small paddock dotted with large black cows. Sue handed me a copy of the weekly itinerary. Each day offered back-to-back activities, including aqua aerobics, bushwalks, life coaching sessions and yoga.

'Don't be intimidated by all the sessions,' Sue reassured me as my eyes scanned the A4 sheet. 'They're all optional. If you'd rather sit by the fire all day and do jigsaw puzzles or read, that's totally fine.'

I spent most of the week alone, exploring the local town and nearby bushland, and drinking herbal teas by the gas fireplace. I did, however, book an appointment with the resident naturopath, Rosemary. I hadn't even mentioned the constant pins-and-needles sensation for her to spot my problem when I sat down in her consultation room. 'You're stressed,' she said bluntly. 'Are you exercising?'

I shook my head guiltily, then told her what was going on with my hands and face.

'The reason that's probably happening is that the hormones your body's making because of the constant stress you're putting it under are building up and manifesting in your extremities. If the stress is going to be constant, then you need to exercise it out of your system,' she said. 'That's going to help, at least in the short term.'

I liked Rosemary's no-nonsense attitude, and what she'd said made complete sense to me. The underlying problems causing the stress, however, needed a different approach, she explained, and she referred me to a psychologist in Sydney to see when I returned home. I did book an appointment with the psychologist, but only attended two sessions. When you're discussing such intimate topics as your own fears, anxieties and problems, a certain level of rapport needs to be established and we simply didn't hit it off.

The numbness had disappeared by the time I stepped back on the train and said goodbye to the tidy, picturesque grounds of Solar Springs. I made a promise to return, before I became a nervous wreck again.

The Name Game

29 June 2016

Dear baby,

We got to see you again today. Our obstetrician's name is Rina, and she will be looking after us over the next eight months to make sure everything is going ok. You looked a bit more like a baby this time when we saw you on the ultrasound. We could see your head and your little limbs, and Rina told us everything looked like it was progressing really well. Your heart's still beating away fast.

Most mums and dads announce they're pregnant after the 12-week scan, and so we've started to tell our close friends and family about you. My belly has begun to swell and it's getting harder and harder to make up excuses as to why I haven't started taking my medicine yet.

Now that you're 12 weeks old in my tummy, I should have stopped worrying that you're going to leave me. You're much stronger now and according to a website I looked at there's a much smaller chance you'll be checking out before we get to meet. But you're not a regular bump, and I'm not your average pregnant woman. So I can't stop thinking you're not going to be there when I wake up each day, and you're too little to give me a kick and let me know you're ok. Now that I've realised I need you more than air, I can't breathe. I won't be able to, until your warm, tiny body is cradled in my arms. I start taking my medicine in a couple of weeks. The doctor says it won't hurt you, but I still don't like the idea of putting a needle in my stomach, so close to you.

There's a chance it will make me feel very sick, and not want to eat. But I will, because I know you need the energy to grow.

You haven't made me feel too sick, so thank you for that. Other mums I know have had a hard time with their little ones in the first trimester, but you've been a dream. I wonder whose personality you're going to have. Will you be chilled and introverted like me, or extroverted, charismatic and fun-loving like your dad? I can't wait to feel you kick.

Much love,
Mum

My mum always said bad things happen in threes. If ever there was a big plane crash on the news, or a celebrity had died, she would say, 'Just you wait, there will be another two. Any day now.'

Cancer happens in threes too, I've come to believe.

'They've found it in my bones,' Dad told me one day in June, just a few weeks after I had told him of my illness. I'd called to check in on him and update him on my pregnancy. He could've told me he'd just had breakfast, such was the casual, unemotional delivery of this devastating news.

It had been a decade since he underwent surgery for his prostate cancer, and he had been monitoring his PSA (prostate-specific antigen) levels every six months since. 'The PSA was a lot higher at the check-up,' he explained, 'so they did a few more tests and the cancer's back. They found a few spots in the bones around my back.'

It had only been a few months since the death of my beautiful cousin, Natalie. She had been battling breast cancer for nearly two decades, and her death had devastated our large family. She was the most beautiful soul, and she had dealt with her illness with such strength right up until her final moments.

'Shit, Dad. Can they treat it? What are they going to do?'

'They're going to try radiation and then put me on hormone therapy,' Dad replied. 'I reckon I've got a few more years, maybe six. I don't want to stick around much longer than that anyway, I'm 70. I've already outlived my father.'

I laughed. I didn't know how else to respond to his dry, sick humour, if that's what it was.

Dad's father died about two years before I was born. My sisters had always spoken so fondly of him, and I always felt sad I never had the chance to meet him. Dad had a painting of him in his study, but the portrait's dark, solemn colours and serious expression used to terrify me as a child. My thoughts wandered to my own baby. Dad had been so happy when we told him we were trying to continue with the pregnancy. He had become soft in his old age, and in recent years had been pushing for Nick and I to hurry up and start a family.

'Well you better stay alive for longer than that, Dad,' I said, 'because you've got another grandchild to spoil for a few more years yet.'

Video diary, 13 July 2016

It's been a while since my last post. I am 14 weeks pregnant now and everything seems to be going really well. I haven't had to have any further tests, the ultrasound for the 12 weeks was really great, they said there were no problems, there were ten fingers and ten toes, so that's been a real relief and a bit of a weight off our chests because it had been a hectic wait. I met with the haematologist again today. I thought I could maybe twist his arm to hold off the interferon treatment which is what I'm going to be taking, because in the last few months my BCR–ABL, which is the marker for the leukaemia I have, has been dropping without me being on any medication. I'd like to think it's because I've been eating really healthily—walking every day and things like that—but we found a report about a woman in Italy whose levels also went down in pregnancy for the whole time she was pregnant, and then they went straight up as soon as she had the baby, so this little person in there seems to be making me healthy! A little miracle baby in more ways than one.

Unfortunately, though, I spoke to Prof today, and despite me bringing this up, he said he'd be much more comfortable with me continuing with the interferon treatment. The side effects sound pretty horrific; fortunately, though, the chemist didn't have the medication to give me, so it's going to start next Sunday. It's a weekly injection and basically creates flu-like symptoms and ruins your desire to eat. Obviously I'm concerned for the baby, so I'm happy I get to wait a little bit longer, because it means I'll be well into the second trimester before I start it.

I feel like a bit of a guinea pig at the moment, because everything's so new and they don't have solid evidence for whether things are good or not for the baby or for me while I'm pregnant, so I'm just trying to give myself the best chance that I can. I'm avoiding too much sugar and just eating a really healthy diet of lots of plant-based foods, and healthy farmed grass-fed beef and proteins, and things like that. It's really all I've got to report. I'm staying really positive. I've had so much support from my family and friends—and yeah, just focusing on feeling better. Hopefully Nick and I are going to go on a little mini break next week because I figured, before I go on the interferon—because I don't know what the next five months are going to bring—it will be nice to spend some quality time together without me feeling like shit before the baby comes, so hopefully that will be nice for just the two of us.

I'll check in with you later . . .

I woke up and mentally scanned my body. My stomach felt ok; no nausea. My body didn't ache, and I wasn't sweaty. My head felt heavy, but there was no pounding or pain, and I didn't feel feverish. I was tired, but hey, I was pregnant, so that was hardly anything new.

I swung my legs over the side of the bed, and slowly stood up.

There was an angry red mark on the right side of my stomach where Nick had administered the first interferon injection the night before. I'd been too scared to do it myself, and Nick had steadier hands. The red welt was the only noticeable side effect of the drug thus far. I walked into the lounge room and gave a little twirl in front of Nick, who was on the couch watching TV.

'I'm ok!' I jumped on top of him and gave him a bear hug. I knew there was a chance the side effects could appear down the track, but so far I was feeling ok.

'Good Ellie,' Nick said. 'I knew you were going to handle it—you're a tough cookie.'

◆ ◆ ◆

We finally managed to organise a weekend away. It had been such an intense few months, and the strain on our relationship was beginning to show. We would get short with each other over the most innocuous things, like which of us forgot to defrost the cat's food, or if we left a plate in the sink for more than a couple of hours.

Being late August it was still bitterly cold, so I suggested making the most of the chilly weather with a three-day stay in the Blue Mountains. 'We could go on bushwalks, eat beautiful food and just enjoy each other's company for a while,' I said. We decided on the newly renovated Hydro Majestic at Medlow Bath. The historic hotel, which was opened in 1904 by retailer Mark Foy, is perched on the edge of a huge escarpment, with incredible views of the Megalong Valley. It's also famed for its ridiculously decadent high tea.

The break turned out to be just the thing we needed. I spent hours each morning walking along the cliff face that ran parallel to the railway, lost in my own thoughts and enjoying the quiet *shhh shhh* of the breeze rustling the towering ghost gums and the crunch of my walking shoes on the wide dirt path.

◆ ◆ ◆

On the second day of our 'babymoon' we spent the afternoon relaxing by the open fire in the hotel lobby, waiting for the sun to set behind the hills surrounding the deep valley. I was engrossed in *Big Little Lies* by author Liane Moriarty when Nick broke the silence.

'If it's a boy, let's call him Thor—like the god of thunder,' he said, staring at the now very obvious bump growing around my middle. I looked up, quizzically, and then smirked, waiting for him to say 'Gotcha!'. It was a game we played, to see which of us was the most gullible. I usually lost, because I am generally more gullible than him—but this time I was sure he was kidding.

'No, you're not going to get me, Nicko, I'm not biting!' I said, shaking my head vehemently.

'I'm dead serious,' he said, trying to repress the beginnings of a smile. 'I think it's a really strong name. We'd pronounce it without the *h* though, so it sounds like *door*, not *thaw*. It's actually the name of a cyclist from Norway who's competing in the Tour de France, Thor Hushovd.'

'I still think you're trying to get me,' I said. 'Besides, I thought we'd decided on Lucky if it was a boy.'

'I think you've been covering celebrities too long, Elle. *Lucky* sounds like something Gwyneth Paltrow would call her kids. He'd get crucified in the playground with a name like that—and you can scrap any notions of him becoming Prime Minister.'

'I think it's really special,' I answered indignantly. 'If everything works out, I'll be the luckiest mum in the world, and he's going to be lucky, too.'

Nick smiled at me. 'Well it's lucky we've got a little while to find something we *both* agree on,' he laughed gently. 'And we've still got to think of a few more girl's names, because there's a fifty per cent chance of that happening too, I guess.'

He gestured to the large window beside the fireplace, which perfectly framed the now orange sun as it dipped behind the mountain range. 'Pretty amazing, huh?' he asked. It was moments like this, I thought, that really made life so worthwhile. The sunset gave way to a deepening blue and for a moment the horizon boasted a pale pink aura. I picked up the drinks menu.

'Alright, well I think baby *Thor* and I should order another peppermint tea before we head to dinner.'

Sharing My Story

Daffodil Day is a charity initiative held every year by the Cancer Council on the fourth Friday of August. It has fallen on my birthday, August 21, once or twice. On the times it did, I loved receiving daffodils as a birthday gift, as they are such a happy-looking bloom, and I knew the money spent was going to a good cause.

In 2016, my awareness of Daffodil Day was much more acute, and it took on a whole new significance for me. About a month prior, I had been sent a media pack with information about the upcoming charity event. I could purchase a pin for $5, the press release told me, or a pin for $2.

I could also share my story, I thought. *Surely that would make a bigger difference to the cause than buying a few pins for my friends and family.* I started workshopping the idea in my head. I considered pitching it as a news story for the paper, but thought twice. Maybe I could just write a piece for online, add a link at the bottom to the charity's website, and it might attract a few extra donations.

If I was going to have leukaemia, I might as well make something positive of it. Lucy Carne, the editor of News Corp's opinion-based Rendezview website, agreed to run a small piece on my experience with CML so far. It took me only about 20 minutes to write the 1200-word story. *I wish I could write fashion and entertainment stories this fast*, I thought once I'd finished. The tears and the emotions I experienced as I summarised the events of the past four months into a few paragraphs proved a surprising release. I felt lighter, somehow, as if the story had been building up in my gut like a wall of little stones, and all of a sudden it had collapsed.

I emailed the copy to Woodsy, my chief of staff, and asked if she would mind having a read. A few minutes later she came over to my desk. 'Hon, I think this would be a great story for the paper,' she said. 'Are you ok if I speak to the team at conference?' Thinking it would warrant a small story on page 30, I agreed.

Later that day, Woodsy told me they were going to run it on Friday. 'We'll need to get a photo of you tomorrow,' she added. 'Can we do the shoot at your home?'

The next day one of the paper's talented young photographers, Dylan Robinson, turned up for what I anticipated would be a quick shoot. The photography team were always extremely efficient. They could shoot bright picture stories in

15 minutes—even less when it came to international celebrities, as a three-minute window was sometimes all the time they were given to nail a shot before the star was whisked off by their minders.

So I was very perplexed that the shoot took more than an hour and a half. Sure, I'm no model, but I've been to enough photo shoots to know how to stand and smile at the camera, and Dylan was a damn good photographer.

Curiously, Dylan wasn't allowed to leave before he'd sent the shots through to the picture desk and had them checked by our editor Chris Dore, or Dorey as he was known. For most shoots, editor approval of photos isn't standard protocol, as the paper's news photographers are among the best in their field, so are generally given plenty of creative scope.

The picture editor called back a few minutes after Dylan sent the shots through. 'He wants more close-up shots,' Dylan said, hanging up the phone. 'And they want you in a different-coloured top.' I changed out of my long-sleeved navy top, into a white silk sleeveless design. We sent through some more shots—and then had to shoot some more. Finally Dylan was allowed to leave.

I felt really happy knowing the story would help raise awareness for a good cause. Most of the stories I wrote for the paper built up or tore down celebrities' egos, or attracted sales for designers or a brand.

I knew my story wasn't going to change the world—or cure cancer for that matter—but it would be a small contribution to the greater good.

Later that day, back in the office, I wandered past the production teams, and saw Dorey and an artist working on what appeared to be the front page. My legs nearly gave way as my eyes scanned down, to see my face plastered across it.

I was tomorrow's front-page splash!

♦ ♦ ♦

After work that evening, I was attending an event for Visit California tourism. Knowing I was going to be on tomorrow's front page, the last thing I wanted to do was mingle. A knot in my stomach twisted tighter and tighter the more I considered the repercussions of my story.

I now regretted putting my personal battle on paper—allowing readers such an intimate peek into my life, and into my head. I was so used to being the vehicle for others to do this, and for the first time I really saw how the subjects of my stories would feel ahead of their own stories appearing in print. It was very confronting.

I wanted to tell Dorey not to run my story so prominently, but I kept reassuring myself that a major news story would undoubtedly break before first edition was printed, relegating mine to a less conspicuous page.

On the way to the event, I called my mum. 'I've written a story for the paper tomorrow on my cancer,' I told her. 'I just wanted to give you the heads up if you get any phone calls from anyone in Sydney, because it probably won't run in *The Courier Mail*.'

'You sound worried. Are you feeling ok?'

'I don't know, Mum. I feel a bit sick. I don't know what the reaction will be like, and I also don't know what's going to happen with the baby. If we lost it, I don't think I could cope if everyone knew what was going on. I'm scared people will think I've made a terrible decision.'

'Everyone's behind you Elle,' she answered. 'Whatever happens, you've done what you thought was best, and that's all you can do. Get some sleep.' She promised to call me in the morning.

The event was a sit-down affair, so I knew I couldn't pull out at such a late stage. I was physically there, but my mind wasn't. I chatted to model and TV presenter Laura Csortan for a while, about pregnancy and babies. She was due to give birth to her first child just a few weeks later. It felt good to talk about pleasant, light-hearted topics, and for a while I forgot about the paper, which by that stage would've been sent to News Corp's printing presses at Chullora. No doubt some breaking news would have bumped me off the front page, in any case.

That night I hardly slept, my mind whirring through all the possible scenarios tomorrow could bring. Earlier that day I had called my friend Alex Needs, the Deputy Executive Producer of Nine's *Today* show, to organise a catch-up with Nick and myself. In passing, I told him I had written a piece for the paper for Daffodil Day.

'We should do something on *Today*,' he'd said to me. 'Would you be keen to come in and have a chat in the morning?'

I said I would. If I was going to share my story, I may as well try and push for as many donations as possible.

Next morning, I got up about 6 a.m. I was too busy preparing for my chat with the *Today* show to check social media or take a quick look at the story online. It was only once I got to Nine's Willoughby studios that I saw my A3-sized face on the front of that day's paper, beside the caption 'Elle's Story'.

◆ ◆ ◆

I didn't really know how I felt, seeing the article. It was a mix of panic, awe and a little bit of pride. I've always been the type of person who prefers to listen, rather than talk. That's what I liked about journalism: I could hear amazing stories, without having to offer up details of my own life. Making myself so vulnerable and exposed had been a very hard thing for me to do.

Nick came along to Nine's studios. I'd been in the cold, cavernous studio countless times, but this time was different. My hands were clammy with sweat and I could feel my heart racing as I was called up to join Lisa Wilkinson, Karl Stefanovic and Sylvia Jeffreys on the desk and share my story with the nation.

The team asked me about my cancer, how I felt when I was first diagnosed, and how people could support further research into the disease. Being able to tell viewers about chronic myeloid leukaemia—an illness I venture had seldom, if ever, been discussed so thoroughly on breakfast TV—was one of the most empowering things I had ever done. I felt so privileged to be able to raise awareness, and encourage Australians to donate money for cancer research. I'd spent years feeling lost and unsure about why I was here on this Earth. I was craving purpose and meaning, and at this moment I finally felt the answer was within my grasp.

As we left the studios, I checked my phone and began to cry. The lock screen was filled with notifications: emails, texts, Instagram likes and Facebook comments. I was stunned.

People I had never met had reached out to offer words of encouragement and support, many also letting me know they had donated or bought a pin in my name.

While all the previous tears I'd shed were borne of sadness and fear, these ones were different. In the space of a few hours, my view of humanity changed. I suddenly felt so connected to every other person and so loved. Years at the newspaper had exposed me to the worst side of humanity—the greed, the corruption, the hatred, the prejudice and the violence. So this new perspective—that people were inherently good, and kind, and loving—felt so uplifting.

On my daily walks I'd been listening to an audio book called *Dying To Be Me*, by Anita Moorjani. The book documented a spiritual awakening Anita had following a near-death experience. She had battled cancer for four years, and when she awoke following her near-death experience her body began to heal in spontaneous remission. 'I realised that the entire universe is composed of unconditional love, and I'm an expression of this,' she writes. 'Every atom, molecule, quark, and tetraquark, is made of love. I can be nothing else, because this is my essence and the nature of the entire universe.'

The words she spoke through my ear buds months before held no meaning at the time. But that day I truly experienced a love beyond my comprehension. The loneliness I had felt since my diagnosis disappeared, replaced by a sense of comfort, and belonging.

◆ ◆ ◆

By the end of the day, my desk at work had disappeared beneath half-a-dozen bunches of flowers. The air in our little showbiz and fashion pod had taken on the sweet scent of freesias and roses. Among the blooms was a bunch of the most flawless cream-coloured roses, wrapped in thick white paper.

'Wanted to let you know I'm thinking of you,' the note read. 'You are strong in soul and spirit; I know you will beat this. Sending love and best wishes and congratulations on your beautiful baby bump. Jen Hawkins x.'

It was such a kind gesture. I have always had a soft spot for Jennifer. I've interviewed her countless times, judged fashion shows with her and witnessed first-hand her decade-long evolution from beauty queen to successful businesswoman. One year prior, Jen had revealed to me that her mum, Gail, had been diagnosed with kidney cancer. She'd received the devastating news just days before she was due to walk the runway for a Myer fashion show, and despite her grief, was honouring her commitment to the retailer she had been the face of for nine years. The day after we broke the story I arrived at the Myer dress rehearsal. I felt awful for Jen and her family, so I stopped by the florist on my way and bought her some flowers. We went through the usual motions, chatting about the upcoming seasonal trends and what we could expect from the summer offering. And while she gave her winning smile and thoughtful responses, I could see she was far from fine. She was heading up to Newcastle after the show, she told me, to be with her family and her mum, who was having surgery that same morning.

Perhaps it was in light of her being touched by cancer so personally that she sent me the beautiful flowers, but whatever her reasons it was a very sweet gesture, and one I'll never forget.

A Mother's Choice

Video diary, 28 August 2016

Seriously, I don't know why I keep doing these videos, and thinking about doing these videos after I've taken all my makeup off. Anyway, it's Sunday night, it's been the biggest weekend of my entire life, tenfold. I still haven't even really processed it and I was thinking about maybe doing a little video on Friday or Saturday, but I've just been so overwhelmed that I haven't been able to.

The emotions that have been rushing through me I've never—you know, felt before so strongly—and I kind of thought it would have passed now, but I actually feel even more emotional because I've had time to let it all sink in.

So on Friday, as a few people know—the readers of The Daily Tele*—I published an article that was going to be a little online piece to celebrate Daffodil Day, but I told my chief of staff that I wanted to write something, and they read the story and they clearly really thought it would resonate with readers, and that afternoon after I filed it I saw the editor working on the front page and my head was on it. That freaked me out, I can't explain to you. I had a little meltdown actually, the night before it came out, thinking Have I done the right thing? Why am I doing this? What's the point? Is it going to mean anything to anybody? And it clearly did to a lot of people, and that was amazing and all of the beautiful messages that I got . . . I just . . . I really don't think that I deserved them, I'm just someone trying to get through every day. I'm feeling really positive and I feel so healthy, which is why I just don't know . . .*

But it's so lovely. But something that really got me as well—the following day when I opened the paper—I didn't know this until I opened the paper, like most readers—was that almost $3 million was donated . . . And I know that wasn't all me, but to know that

I played a small part, it made me feel like my life was really worth living and, like I'd done something to give back, and I think my little baby would be proud of me. . . Sorry, I didn't think I'd get so emotional doing this video.

Anyway the whole thing was really surreal. Oh, I just felt him kicking, haha—that was kind of cool!

I have my next appointment at the RPA on Thursday at the Women and Babies hospital. So I guess I'll just look at the ultrasound and check that everything's ok. They'll probably ask me a few questions about the story, because I didn't think it was going to be anything big, so I didn't really, you know, get in touch with anyone about it to let them know, or give them the heads up, so I have a feeling my haematologist will be asking me a few questions when I see him next.

Anyway I guess I just wanted to, I don't know, get all of that off my chest, and lodge this video so I'll always remember how amazing the last 48 hours were, and how grateful I am that all of these beautiful people from my childhood have come out, and strangers I've never met have given me prayers and are sending me and my family so much love. It's been life-changing—more than even, you know, all the stuff that's happened to me. This has made more of an impact in my life than anything. So I just wanted to—this probably won't ever see the light of day—but I wanted to express my gratitude and have this as a memento of a beautiful time.

That night, as I turned off the lights in the lounge room and made my way to bed, I felt calm. I had thousands of people sending me good vibes, and prayers. And in that moment I loved them. I loved every single one of them with every inch of my being, for loving me, and my baby. The anger and fear that had been following me around like shadows felt less present.

A peace had washed over me; a sense that everything was going to work out ok.

I looked down at my stomach, which by now had partially obstructed my view of my feet. 'I hope you're proud of me, little boy,' I whispered to my unborn son, and crept into bed.

We had found out our baby's gender just a few days before Daffodil Day. At our 19-week scan, we asked the sonographer if he would mind sending a secret text to the owner of our favourite cake shop in Canterbury, telling her, but not *us*, our baby's sex, so she could get to work on a gender-reveal cake.

'Can you definitely tell if it's a boy or a girl?' Nick asked the sonographer. 'Because, you know, we don't want to cut open a cake and see pink *and* blue!'

The sonographer laughed. 'No, I'm pretty positive of the sex.'

We asked him to delete the text as soon as he'd sent it, so we had absolutely no way of finding out if we were having a boy or girl.

The 'gender reveal' has only become popular in the past few years. Rather than find out in the ultrasound room, or on the day of the birth, a growing number of expectant couples are making the gender reveal into a celebration of its own. They will give a cake shop an envelope containing a note with their unborn baby's sex, and the baker will then create a blue- or pink-layer cake, encased in a thick layer of white icing. Some couples use boxes filled with pink or blue balloons, and I've even heard of gender-reveal piñatas.

Nick and I decided to combine our gender reveal with my birthday, on August 21. The cake would reveal the sex of our baby, and double as my birthday cake. We had our families over for dinner, and arranged Skype calls with my sisters and nephews in Brisbane so we could all find out together. Everyone was taking bets on the gender. I predicted we were having a boy; Nick thought it would be a girl, as did my sisters and his parents.

After dinner I blew out the candles on the cake, took Nick's hand, and together we slowly sliced down the centre of the towering white dessert, creating a thick wedge with two knives. We slid the large slice gingerly towards ourselves, then lifted it up.

'It's a BOY!!!' we shouted as we saw the unmistakeable royal-blue hue sandwiched between two fluffy chunks of butter cake.

Everybody was cheering and hugging, and there were a few tears.

It was the first time Nick and I had allowed ourselves to celebrate, and enjoy, the miracle we had made together. We didn't care if we had a boy or a girl. We just wanted a healthy baby, but being able to talk to him, and imagine a future with our little boy in it, felt so unbelievably special. It was a moment I'll never forget.

Had our circumstances been different, we would have considered not finding out until the day of the birth. But unlike most couples, our entry into parenthood was far from joyous. I felt robbed of the excitement we should have felt when we first saw the positive pregnancy test. If only I'd taken it a couple of days earlier, we would've at least been able to celebrate briefly, before my cancer diagnosis brought us crashing back down to earth.

In those early weeks, an emotional tug-of-war took place inside my head every time I thought about my unborn baby—my feelings of excitement ripped away by panic and despair. I tried so hard not to let the negative emotions win, but any happy thoughts I had were tainted.

A Mother's Choice

By mid-August, however, the apprehension had begun to dim, replaced by a growing sense of hope. My BCR–ABL levels were steady, and we were only a few weeks away from hitting the 26-week gestation mark. The survival rate of premature babies significantly increases in those born after 26 weeks. By 32 weeks, the likelihood of survival is almost in line with babies born full term.

If I could make it through the next month and a half without my cancer levels spiking, there was a chance we would both survive this.

I was counting down the days.

Video diary, 14 September 2016

Just outside getting my daily vitamin D dose. I've heard it's not only good for your baby but also for cancer, so that's what I'm doing today. I got some more results back this week after visiting the haematologist, which was my BCR–ABL (cancer gene) levels. I'm a little bit disappointed because the first time I got them checked, they had gone down from 18 per cent to 15 per cent, which is a really good result, and I was really hopeful that they'd go down again. But they haven't, they're still at 15 per cent—which isn't necessarily a bad thing according to my haematologist, but it just means that because I've been tolerating the interferon medication so well, he's asked me to double the dosage, so I'll start that this week. I'm a little bit nervous about that but hopefully I will be a cancer unicorn and not have any side effects, fingers crossed . . .

The cat has just run into the bushes, nowhere to be found . . .

Anyway, so yeah, just trying to eat really healthy; I went to prenatal yoga this morning, which was really good for my mental health as well. I got some bad news about my dad: he's got prostate cancer and he's found out it's spread to his bones, which is pretty upsetting—and one of my husband's mates died of leukaemia last weekend, so I'm really hoping I win the Lotto because I really feel like I—well, me and my husband—need some good luck.

Actually Nick has had to deal with so much, and I'm so grateful to have him in my life, because he's just been everything to me. He's my rock, so I hope something good happens to him in the next few weeks because he deserves it.

I have my ultrasound on Thursday, so hopefully bub is tracking well. He's kicking like a maniac, which is a really good sign, and I'm still gaining weight which is good, so yeah. Just enjoying the sunshine, and trying to stay positive.

Speak soon.

In early October I returned to Solar Springs. I was becoming extremely fatigued and felt like I needed a break from my life. I wanted a week to myself, without hearing the words *leukaemia* or *cancer*.

I just wanted to be a heavily pregnant woman in need of a pedicure and some hours by a fireplace.

After a brave, four-year battle with acute leukaemia, Nick's school friend had tragically passed away. While Nick did his best to keep his emotions in check in front of me, I could tell the news had hit him hard. It was a sobering reminder that despite having navigated the past few months without any major developments in my illness, cancer was an unpredictable disease with no master.

The moment I walked into the cosy foyer, with its blond-wood reception desk and dark 80s-era carpet, I felt like

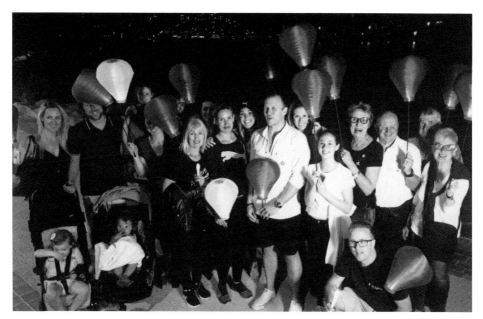

October 2016. Taking part in the Leukaemia Foundation's Light the Night event at Barangaroo with friends and family. Despite the frequent tears, we all had such a wonderful time and raised a lot of money.

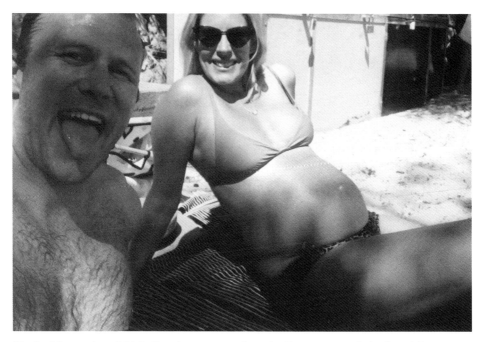

Early November 2016. Getting some vitamin D one month before Tor was born. We enjoyed one last babymoon at the Watson's Bay Hotel on the weekend of our wedding anniversary.

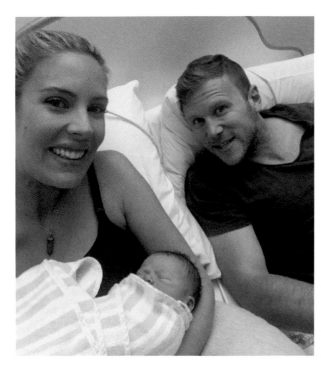

The day after Tor was born. I'm still wearing my lucky bloodstone necklace.

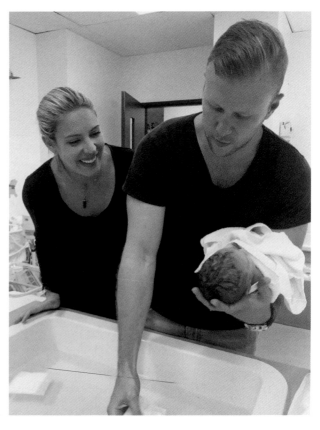

Giving Tor his first bath.

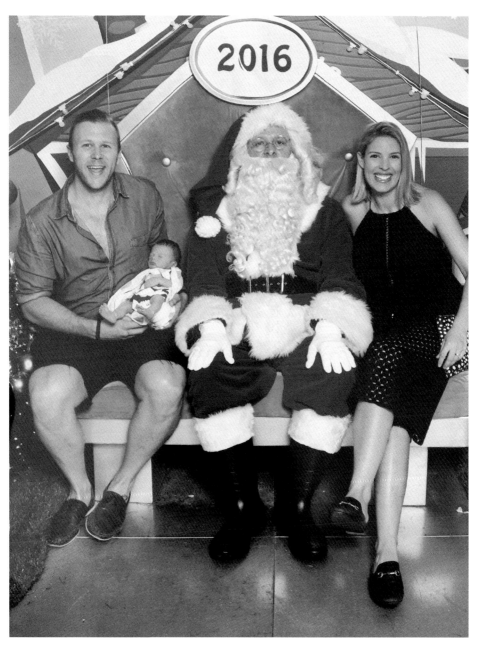

Our first family Santa photo! Tor was only about ten days old here.

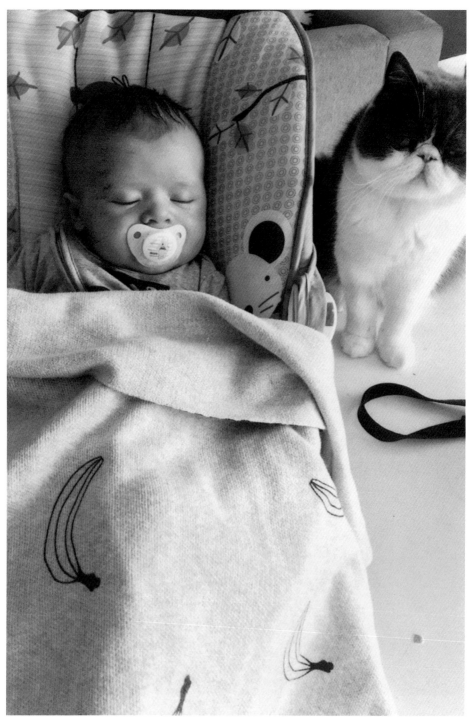

Chairman Meow was not so sure about his new brother, who smelled like milk and looked nothing like him.

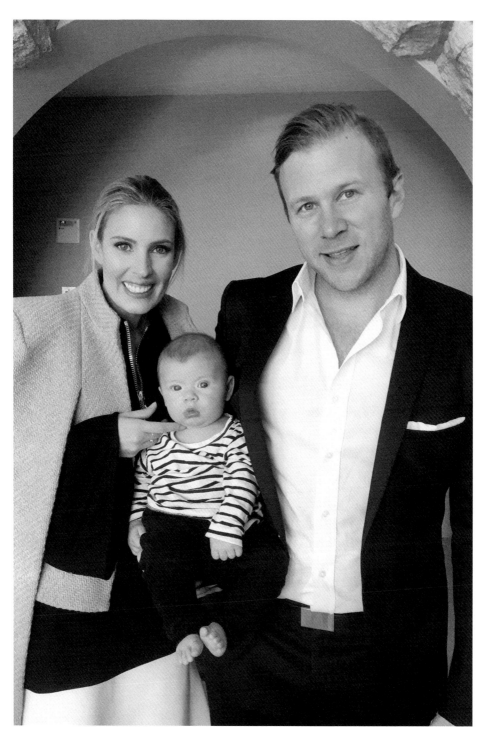

This pic was taken the week of my first cancerversary in April 2017. It was a very bittersweet time but we were on our way to my cousin's wedding and I was feeling really positive that day.

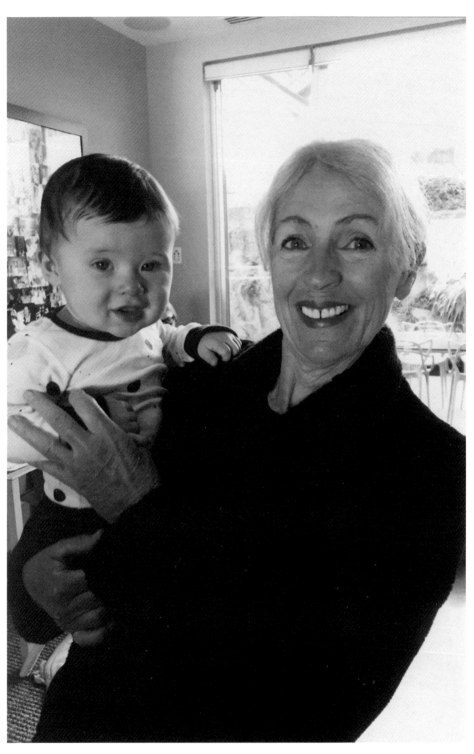

My mum and Tor in August 2017. Mum lives in Brisbane but came to Sydney for two weeks to help look after him.

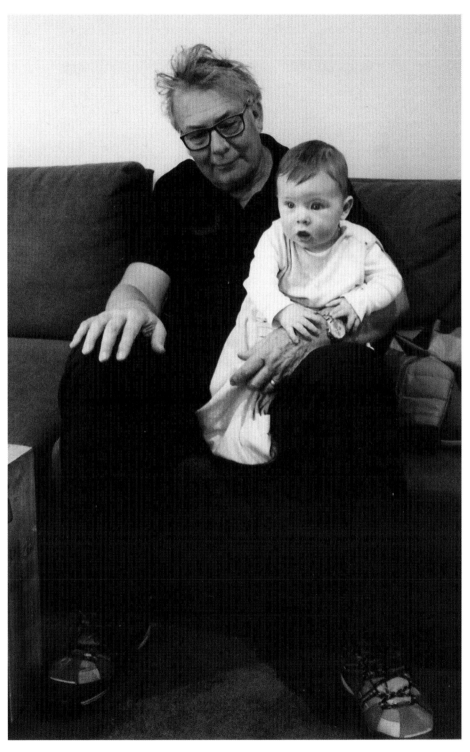

Dad and Tor on a family snow trip to Thredbo that same month.

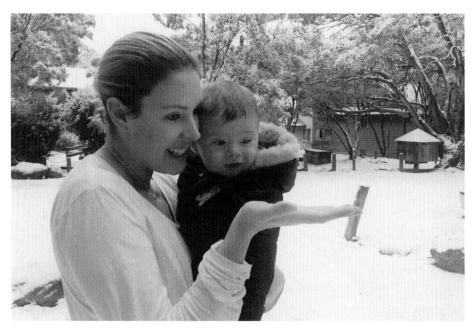

Tor experiencing snow for the first time. He loved the cold weather and was spoiled rotten by his nephews, aunties and uncles and Dad and Dad's wife Suzette on the trip.

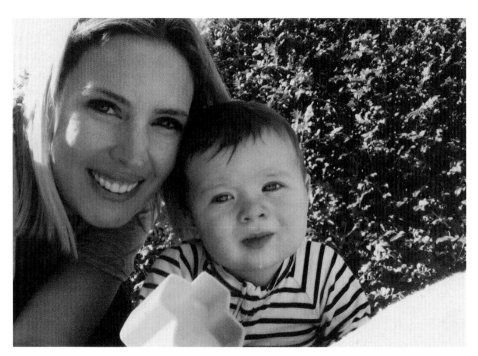

My favourite kind of days involve playing in the backyard with Tor, pointing at the planes. I couldn't ask for anything better.

I was home again. I lugged my small suitcase to my room, and plonked my heavy body on the bed. I was starting to crave the feeling of lying on my stomach, having been unable to for the past four months. I bemoaned the fact I hadn't been able to book a room with an ensuite this time, considering my bladder now felt about the size of a small ice cube.

I let the manager know of my illness, but after a few days at the retreat my fellow guests simply thought of me as 'the pregnant lady'. It felt great answering questions about the gender, baby names and how much longer I had to go, rather than how my treatment was going.

Every day I spent meditating, sketching, and wandering the retreat's beautifully manicured grounds, and reflecting on the past year of my life and how much it had changed.

Video diary, 7 October 2016

I am feeling so amazing; relaxed and happy. I just finished five nights at Solar Springs health retreat. It's the second time I've been here. I came here about 18 months ago because I was feeling a bit stressed from work, so I thought it would be nice to have a little solo baby-moon for a few nights, and it's been so beneficial. I feel so renewed. I read some novels, and got a massage and treatments and went for beautiful walks around the bushland. It's such a beautiful spot here in Bundanoon. Everything's just quaint and quiet and you wake up to the birds . . .

Health-wise I'm feeling pretty good. Tired. But I can't complain. When you get up and you can stand up out of bed and go for a walk, how can you feel bad? I just am really grateful that I can still do those things, and so I'm going to make the most of it and take as much advantage of that as I can, because I know that I'm very lucky to be in this situation right now.

So gratitude I guess is the main thing for me right now, and I'm just really grateful that the pregnancy is going so smoothly.

Only one more trimester to go; I'm just about to hit the third trimester.

Ok, bye.

Every month or so I would receive a call from a representative from the Leukaemia Foundation, to check how I was doing. It was so nice to have someone check in occasionally who knew what questions to ask, and could also answer queries I had about my disease and how to deal with it from a lifestyle perspective.

A few weeks after my story appeared in *The Telegraph* I received a flyer from the Foundation, calling on Australians to take part in Light The Night, their annual fundraising walk. On an evening in October, people with leukaemia and their loved ones were invited to walk together with a lantern in hand to raise funds for research into blood cancer and to support sufferers.

Nick suggested we get a group together for the walk. He can attest that while I am reasonably organised when it comes to my job, my social life is a shambles. I would forget my own birthday if Facebook didn't remind me. I think I got that unfortunate trait from my dad, who can be a little absent-minded. He's pretty much a genius when it comes to fixing engines and anything with a motor, but if he didn't have his wife Suzette around, I think he'd forget to eat.

In fact, one year Dad gave me a birthday card emblazoned with the words 'You're *how* old?!' on the front. He actually had no clue how old I was. I didn't hold it against him, though, because despite being forty years younger than him I'm still just as bad.

I write everything down, and I mean *everything* when it comes to organising myself for work, and by the time the weekend rolls around my mental capacity for organising catch-ups with friends and family has usually been exhausted, so I leave everything to Nick. He's much more enthusiastic about socialising, so I let him take charge of our events calendar.

So as usual, the week of the event rolled around and I still hadn't told a single person about it. Fortunately, while I dithered and procrastinated, Nick had invited a few mates and our families to take part, so on 7 October we had a group of more than twenty join us at Barangaroo on Sydney Harbour for the walk.

A few days after my story in *The Daily Telegraph*, Stef, a producer from Nine's *60 Minutes* program, contacted me. She asked if Nick and I would be willing to be interviewed about my cancer and pregnancy for the current affairs show. In return, the show would donate to a charity of my choosing.

After about a week of persuasion, Nick finally agreed. He's a very private person and had reservations about appearing on national television. I thought it was a great opportunity to spread awareness of chronic myeloid leukaemia, as so few people had even heard of the illness, and I felt somewhat obliged to use my position in the media to draw attention to it. Reporter Allison Langdon would do the interview, Stef explained; Allison was also pregnant, and was due to give birth just a few days after me, so it would tie in nicely.

On the evening of Light The Night, Ally, Stef and the production crew also joined our walking party, to film the event for the story.

My mum had set up a fundraising page on the charity's website a few weeks beforehand, and managed to raise an impressive $5000 ahead of the event. She was one of their top individual fundraisers, and her name appeared on the outdoor screen that was set up at the starting point. I was so proud of her.

When the sun finally set, the crowd of two thousand participants flicked on their lanterns. There were three different-coloured lanterns, each with a special meaning. Blue lanterns were held by those supporting someone they knew with blood cancer, yellow lanterns were lit in honour of loved ones who had passed away from the illness, while survivors or people currently fighting the disease carried white lanterns.

I stepped away from the group for a moment to take in the sunset and watch as dozens, then scores, and finally hundreds of coloured lights began to illuminate the waterfront park. It was an awe-inspiring sight. I flicked on the switch of my white lantern, and looked around at the glowing sea of blue, punctuated by points of yellow, and white. As I gazed at each of those white lanterns, I felt the isolation of my illness drop away. *Each person holding a white lantern*, I thought, *has a story like mine*. I wanted to approach every single one of those lantern holders and hug them. I wanted to know their stories, and gain strength from them. I wanted to share in their sorrow, their grief and their hope.

I wondered how a representation of blood cancer—an illness that devastated children, siblings, parents and partners—could look so beautiful. But it was. The sight of thousands of illuminated orbs as they began their journey around the water's edge was stunning.

I rejoined my friends and family, and we melted into the huge procession as it meandered slowly around the waterfront. I smiled as my small, white light became surrounded by a reassuring ring of blue, and took comfort in the knowledge that I need never feel alone.

◆ ◆ ◆

What's 'hard' about it? Save your own life. Why risk two lives to try and make some stupid point?

Just minutes after my *60 Minutes* story aired, the show's Facebook page had lit up with dozens of comments from viewers.

Life can be so cruel at times . . . Dear God please help this family, one of the comments read.

Hang in there Elle, wrote another.

Dozens wrote that they were praying everything worked out, and sent words of encouragement and kindness.

Most were wholeheartedly supportive, but a few took umbrage with my choice to keep my baby.

I was labelled 'selfish', 'reckless' and a bad mother for bringing a child into the world considering there was a chance my illness could progress and kill me. Some people thought the idea of leaving my baby motherless was akin to child abuse. Others praised me for putting the life of my unborn baby first, and some openly wondered what they would do in my situation. One or two even advised me to give medical marijuana a whirl, which would cure me in no time. Uh-huh.

In fact, a few had offered up their opinions on the social media page even before the show aired, based on the brief promo ads which had begun running earlier that week.

I could imagine how upsetting those comments could be, had I not become desensitised to them. Mum found it hard, and began responding to the haters in my defence. 'Mum, please don't write any more replies to people posting negative comments,' I texted after seeing her name appear in the feed. 'It just eggs them on. I'm not bothered by them, honestly.'

Perhaps I'd have felt differently if the story had aired earlier on in my pregnancy—but having weathered the first and second trimesters, and being less than two months from my due date, I felt like I had made the right choice for myself and our family.

Every kick I felt, and every time I saw my baby boy on the ultrasound screen, reinforced my decision. There was already nothing I wouldn't do to protect him.

So Close

As the chilly days of winter finally gave way to the warmer days of spring, life settled into a rhythm of doctor's appointments, work and long walks. I began taking on more work as my energy increased, and was soon back covering events for the paper and contributing fashion stories to Sydney Confidential and the Saturday *Daily Telegraph*.

It was strange bumping into industry contacts I hadn't spoken to since the diagnosis. Their faces would contort with different emotions as they struggled to know what to say. It generally went something like this:

'Hi [insert publicist/agent/celebrity], nice to see you,' I'd say.

'How are you, Elle?' they would reply automatically, before pausing and wondering if they'd opened up a can of worms by asking about my wellbeing. 'I mean, obviously you're not alright, but—' they would add, looking slightly embarrassed, '—but you look great!'

Then they'd spy my pregnant stomach and exclaim 'Oh and. . . congratulations?' The comment ended with an upwards inflection, as if to ask whether the pregnancy was indeed something to congratulate me on.

A lot of people found it hard to know what to say, and I understood. If someone had said to me, 'Wow, you've had a really shitty run, haven't you? Glad it's not me. Anyway, I really hope you don't die,' with sincerity, I wouldn't have been upset. I discovered very quickly that cancer made people feel very uncomfortable. One friend disappeared from my life almost immediately after I told him about my diagnosis. When we ran into each other a few months later, he acted as if nothing had happened. 'Hey, great to see you,' he said, walking off before I could even respond. That was it. Not even a text afterwards to ask about my health, or how I was doing, or to apologise for the radio silence. I don't blame him, but it was a shock as most of my friends had been incredibly supportive.

The weekly injections were still tolerable, despite Prof doubling my dose in recent weeks, thanks to my ability to tolerate the drug without major side effects. Not that I was completely symptom free. I struggled some days to get out of bed, and walking up a flight of stairs felt like scaling Everest. However,

I was feeling more and more upbeat as the pregnancy continued, with my due date crawling closer and closer. I was having my blood taken every few weeks, checking that the cancer markers were still stable. My BCR–ABL score had recently jumped from about nine per cent to the mid teens, which wasn't ideal but not alarming.

I was almost part of the furniture at the Royal Prince Alfred. I spent hours each week in the waiting room at the Lifehouse or Women and Babies department. On at least three occasions I arrived at the haematology department, only to be informed I wasn't expected that day, so I'd rush to the maternity ward and sure enough, I'd be due there for a scan or check-up instead.

◆ ◆ ◆

On 28 November, I had an appointment with Prof. The latest tests revealed my cancer marker had jumped to 18 per cent. It was trending upwards despite the weekly interferon injections. 'It shows we don't have complete control of the disease,' Prof explained.

He told me not to worry, which was easier said than done. Fortunately I was now 34 weeks pregnant, and had reached the point where my baby could be induced and have an extremely good chance of survival—but now the question was whether my decision to delay treatment could affect the possibility that I would reach a full remission on the drugs after the baby was born. I had no choice but to wait and see.

The original plan was to induce me at 38 weeks if everything was going smoothly, but my obstetrician Rina had suggested 36 weeks would also be fine if my health took a turn.

I didn't want to risk my cancer level increasing, so after consulting with Rina it was decided I would be induced in two weeks time.

29 November 2016

Dear Baby,
Looks like you're going to be a Sagittarian, not a Capricorn. The doctors have given you a birthday: December 13, 2016, four weeks earlier than your expected due date. Dad is happy as he was a bit worried you'd arrive on Christmas Day, which, he thinks, would be the worst thing ever for a kid because it would steal all your thunder. But really, we wouldn't care what day you were born, because we would both make sure you always felt super special and would just be happy to have you with us.

Rina says you are growing very fast, and are in the 99th percentile for weight, so hopefully you'll be big and strong enough to handle coming into the world a little undercooked. I've been stuffing my face with salmon and avocado in the hope I can pad you out a bit before you arrive. You also have a very big head, which is a bit worrying; I hope we can get you out without too much drama.

I wish we could give you a beautiful nursery filled with toys and pretty things, but we live in a small, one-bedroom apartment so you'll have to make do bunking with us in our room. It's cosy. I have bought you your own chest of drawers, though.

On Sunday your aunty Christina threw us both the most beautiful baby shower ever. We ate cucumber sandwiches, played games and I even treated myself to a homemade vanilla cupcake (which tasted like heaven). My friends and family showered you with the most wonderful gifts—soft pastel bunnies, train sets, books, soft swaddles and onesies

in grey, white and blue. I've washed and folded them neatly in your
drawers, and next week Dad will put together your bassinet.

We're nearly ready to meet you. Hang in there.

All my love,

Mum

The evening before I was admitted to the hospital, Nick and I drove down to Bondi Beach for a swim. I had become obsessive about getting lots of vitamin D throughout my pregnancy, and thus had a very enviable tan. I looked pretty healthy, and very pregnant. We wandered along the promenade and down onto the sand of North Bondi. The beach resembled a giant infinity pool; there was little in the way of a swell, save for a delicately ebbing and flowing shoreline beckoning beachgoers into its calm waters.

Nick and I shook out our towels and lay down, taking in the last warmth of the day's sun.

'I'm so proud of you, Elle,' Nick said after a while. 'You don't complain; you just get on with things, even though you absolutely have the right to yell and scream and say how unfair everything is. You know you can—you don't have to be brave around me.'

'I'm scared,' I told him, after a few moments' silence. 'I'm scared about tomorrow, and how it's going to play out—and I'm also scared about becoming a mum. But there's no point wallowing in self-pity and letting my fear get the better of me. It's only going to make me feel worse.'

I paused. 'You know, if someone told me they could wipe the events of the past year away, and cure my leukaemia and make this a run-of-the-mill pregnancy, I don't think I would have asked them to. I'm such a different person to who I was before this happened, and I think it's for the better.'

If the drugs didn't work, and my life did begin drifting away, my only regret would be for my son. I would rob him of a mother, and leave Nick to pick up the pieces of a family made whole for just a few, fleeting moments.

I felt I had begun to know myself for the first time in these past eight months. Cancer had peeled back the superficial layers which I had created over the years, and I finally saw myself as I truly was. And I liked that person much more. She was kinder, more vulnerable, more soft. But she was also fierce, powerful and fearless. She was love.

◆ ◆ ◆

I stood up, walked to the shore and waded into the surf, letting the crisp, cool ocean water envelop my warm, pregnant belly for the final time. I was hoping to give birth vaginally, but knew many induced births ended in C-sections, so I'd been mentally preparing for both scenarios.

All the books I'd read stressed expectant mothers should have a birth plan, outlining if they wanted pain relief or an epidural, and if they wanted a water birth or a conventional, hospital-bed type. But this pregnancy had begun in the most unusual of circumstances, so I knew anything could happen, and I simply had to go with the flow.

I had begun expressing colostrum two days beforehand, in the hope of storing a few millilitres of the nutritious pre-milk to give the baby. The tyrosine kinase inhibitor drugs were too dangerous to take while breastfeeding, so I had allowed myself just a week to give him my colostrum before starting them and stopping the interferon injections. I wanted to give my son the best start to his life that I could, and if that meant holding off my own life-giving treatment for a few days, then so be it.

I had been researching breast milk donation banks ahead of the birth in the hope of supplementing formula with human breast milk, but I soon realised how hard it was to access it unless you had a very premature baby. It was quite disheartening, with my only option to fork out a ridiculous amount of money—approximately $1 per mL—or post an ad on Facebook. I would need to see medical records and be extremely comfortable with the woman who was willing to provide it if I went down the latter route.

But in an incredibly selfless act, a family friend of Nick's parents reached out, letting me know their daughter Jade had an oversupply and would be willing to donate her excess milk if I needed it.

That gesture made my heart soar, and I'll be forever grateful to Jade for giving me a chance to feed my baby breast milk for a few weeks longer than I was able.

I dunked my head beneath the water, then lay on my back. I floated silently, watching the last light of the summer evening slowly dim, replaced by the indigo night. I felt so peaceful, and so grateful at that moment. That I had made it this far, and that in the next 48 hours I would meet my brave, strong son.

Baby Tor

17 December 2016

Dear Baby Tor,

My heart is as big as a blimp. You have arrived, and you are perfect. You have brown hair, full pillow lips and ten fingers and ten toes. Your eyes are dark, but I think they might end up a bright blue, like your dad's.

We hope you like your name, Tor. It's Scandinavian and means 'god of thunder'. It also means 'craggy hill' in Scottish, but trust us, that wasn't the inspiration. Tor is a strong name, just like you. Your middle name is Felix, which is the Latin word for 'lucky'.

A Mother's Choice

I've hardly slept these past four days. It's not just because you're keeping me awake. I'm scared that if I shut my eyes even for the briefest of moments you'll disappear, like a little ghost.

Dad celebrated your arrival with pizza. He had a barbecue-chicken thin base delivered to the birthing suite an hour after you arrived, much to the shock of the delivery driver. Dad stashed the half-empty box beneath your portable crib, which we walked upstairs to our room, and I couldn't stop giggling, even though I was ridiculously exhausted after an eight-hour labour, and my now soft, inflated tummy was spasming with pain each time I did.

You have had so many visitors, and everyone who has met you says you look just like your dad. Your aunty Sandy knitted you the most beautiful blue booties and sent a giant blue bear with a balloon, just for you. You're going to have trouble deciding on a favourite toy, or book for that matter, because you have been blessed with so many from your new family and friends.

I'm deliriously happy, but I also feel sick with guilt. I'm ashamed I even entertained the idea that I had a choice, because I didn't. You needed to be here, on this earth, with me.

I don't know what the next few months will bring. The medicine I need to take might make me feel yucky, but it won't matter, as long as it's working and I get to be with you.

You won't get to read this for a long time, but I have set you up with your very own email address so that me and your aunties, uncles and grandparents can tell you how much we adore you.

We get to take you home tomorrow, baby Tor.

Welcome to the world.

Love, Mum

Sydney was in the midst of a heatwave the week Tor came into our lives. The temperature in the Royal Prince Alfred Hospital's maternity ward, however, was a pleasant 22 degrees. I had neither the energy, nor the desire, to leave the comfortably cool hospital in the days after the birth. In fact, I didn't venture further than the kitchen down the hall, which I'd visit every afternoon to fetch one of the half-dozen organic orange and mango ice blocks Mum had scoured half of Sydney's organic supermarkets to track down for me.

Nick was in complete awe of Tor. It took us about two days to officially name him, but we already knew him as Tor, or by his affectionate nickname Tormy. The panic I had felt in the days leading up to the birth had dissolved, replaced by new fears. Every time I looked at his tiny pink features I felt a surge of heat rush through me. *Here you are, perfect in every way,* I thought to myself, *but surely this can't last. I can't be that lucky.* I felt an immense pressure and responsibility to never let anything harm him.

'Nothing can prepare you for fatherhood, son,' Nick's dad had told him a few days before the birth. He was so right, as neither of us could have anticipated the waves of emotions that ebbed and flowed through us both in the following days. My illness became totally insignificant at that point. What had just a week ago dominated my thoughts now barely registered, as the schedule of feeding, bathing, and the constant stream of visitors took up my time and energy. It was a blissful reprieve, allowing me to immerse myself in the crazy but beautiful world of motherhood.

It was during Tor's first bathtime that I really had the chance to witness Nick's growing bond with our son. We were both so nervous as we wheeled him into the warm bathing room. It took an eternity for Nick to pull off Tor's tiny newborn-sized singlet and place him in the shallow bath, watching his tiny body react to the warm water's embrace. It was at this moment, as I watched Nick washing our son with such incredible care, that I realised what a wonderful dad he would be. His face was a mix of worried concentration and disbelief at what we had created, and my heart could not have been filled with more love as I watched on.

About two days into my new role as a mum, J.Mo and Briana came to visit. They were planning to run a story alerting the paper's readers to Tor's arrival, and it proved a good excuse for the pair to meet him.

Having my photo taken was the last thing I felt like doing, and I really wanted to just hibernate with my new family—but having worked at the paper for a decade, and considering the overwhelming support I received from both my colleagues and *The Daily Telegraph*'s readers when I told them of my ordeal, I felt compelled to share our joy with them.

The next day, at about 7 a.m, I dragged my aching body out of bed, determined to leave the maternity ward and feel some fresh air on my face. I was hit with an overwhelming sense of joy as I walked out of the hospital's main entrance and felt the sun's warm rays touch my skin. It was instantly energising. Despite the muscle pains, sore breasts and my looming cancer battle, I felt invincible.

A New Challenge

A week after the birth, I received a call from Prof's registrar. He had the results from my latest blood test.

'Your BCR–ABL has dropped from 21 per cent to 9 per cent,' Prof's registrar confirmed.

I couldn't believe it. It had been climbing steadily in the final weeks of the pregnancy, despite the weekly interferon injections. The registrar explained that this sudden drop may have been a delayed response to the interferon injections.

I hung up the phone and put my head in my hands. The relief caused a flood of fresh tears, not my first for the day. Nick thought I'd been given bad news.

'It's not bad,' I managed to say. 'It's good. *Really* good. My levels have plummeted below 10 per cent.'

I decided to breastfeed for another month. It wasn't something my doctors would have advised, but I'd gotten this far without the drugs, so a few more weeks couldn't hurt, surely.

The birth had been uncomplicated. I had been induced, and aside from the first epidural not working, everything had run smoothly. I hadn't needed a C-section, and despite his four-week prematurity Tor had been born weighing a healthy 3.1 kg and needed no time in the special care nursery.

It was an extremely uneventful end to the most complicated year of my life. But I knew my battle was still far from over.

◆ ◆ ◆

A few days after we arrived home, our life settled into a cycle of feeding, nappy changing and short bursts of sleep. Tor was an easy baby, but the lack of sleep and the magnitude of the next phase of my cancer battle, which involved starting the tyrosine kinase inhibitor drugs and coping with whatever side effects they caused, had begun to affect me mentally.

I hoped that, like the interferon, my body would cope with the chemical onslaught and I'd experience few, if any, severe symptoms, but the drugs affected every person differently so it was impossible to know. On the rare occasions that I had a moment to myself, I would sit quietly and visualise myself taking the twice-daily medication and feeling absolutely fine. I had no idea if it would help in any way, but it helped me to keep my worry in check.

Tor was just shy of two weeks old when Christmas rolled around. Nick's family and mine were big on celebrating the festive season. Nick's sister Chrissy and I would blast Mariah Carey's hit 'All I Want For Christmas' at every opportunity from mid-November, and the decorations went up as soon as it was reasonably acceptable.

But yuletide shenanigans were the furthest thing from my mind in the days after Tor's birth. I managed to scrape myself together enough on Christmas Eve to get our very first family Christmas photo. We only lived about 100 metres from Birkenhead Point shopping centre, so it was an easy stroll down. I'd dressed Tor in a cute, kitsch, red-and-white onesie emblazoned with a reindeer head decal, and thrown on a pair of navy culottes and a matching top. We stuck the overpriced Santa photos on the fridge when we got home, and I collapsed on the couch, knackered.

◆ ◆ ◆

Shelley Bell had warned me about this during one of our first conversations. 'You'll probably be quite sensitive in those first weeks after the birth,' she said. 'You've just spent those first months concentrating on getting through the pregnancy, but then once it's time to focus on you and your own health, it can be pretty confronting.'

She was right. I spent nights wiping tears from Tor's head as they dripped down my face during feeds. I kept thinking back to my life a year before. My uncomplicated, baby-free, cancer-free and somewhat carefree life. I felt like a zombie, walking around in a state of half-wakefulness and half-sleep. I dreaded the thought of anybody visiting, and had warned Nick that I would need time alone to adjust to life as a new mum. But we still had what felt like a revolving door of friends and family dropping in to see how we were doing. It was super nice, and we really appreciated the support, but it was exhausting.

I quickly perfected a response to questions. If I stuck to my mentally rehearsed script, I could cope. 'He's a great baby,' I'd say, with a smile. 'Yes, I'm getting a little sleep. Feeling a bit tired, but otherwise really good. We're so lucky having Nick's parents and my mum here for support; they've been amazing. Yeah I start treatment in February. I'll be on the drugs indefinitely at this stage. We'd like more kids but we're not sure if we'll be able to. It depends on my response to the treatment—but we're so happy with one.'

If anyone had gone off-script, had dug further into how I was really coping post-birth and pre-treatment, the facade may have cracked.

Eating had suddenly dropped to the bottom of my priority list. After eight months spent obsessing over every single mouthful of food, I had no energy to even *think* about meals. Instead, I adopted an iced coffee diet, which would involve downing two 500 mL bottles of the caffeinated liquid between 5.30 a.m. and 3 p.m. and then praying I'd be able to get some form of sleep that night. I can't imagine what a shock it was to my body, which I'd treated so well for the best part of the year. It had carried my son and delivered him safely despite its poor state of health, and now I was treating it like a rubbish bin.

Nick would often walk in and find me crying. 'I'm just so tired,' I'd wail. I couldn't believe the effect lack of sleep had on my mind. I felt permanently jet-lagged, and even the most inane, unimportant thoughts would send me into fits of sobbing.

Paranoia about sudden infant death syndrome also constantly assailed my thoughts. While there was no definitive evidence of a genetic disposition, having lost my big brother, Eric, to SIDS had made me extremely panicky about bedtime. I'd wake up in the middle of the night, and if I couldn't hear any breathing I'd jump out of bed, rush over to Tor's cot and put my ear to his mouth to make sure he still was.

My illness had taken up so much of my time during the pregnancy that I'd had little opportunity to think about how motherhood itself would impact my life. Having cancer was hard, but having cancer and being a new mum was fucking brutal.

◆ ◆ ◆

I googled *postnatal depression* more than once in those first few weeks.

I've been able to laugh and see the funny side of things, read the first statement in the 'Do You Have Postnatal Depression Quiz'. I'd chuckled when Tor had peed all over Nick's T-shirt the day before, so I ticked *Sometimes*.

I ticked *Quite often* for the statements *I've been so unhappy that I've been crying*, and *I've been anxious or worried for no good reason*. But then I told myself that having leukaemia exempted me from the latter question, as I had a totally good reason to be anxious and worried, so I downgraded my response to *Sometimes*.

'It's possible that you do have postnatal depression,' the quiz concluded anyway.

I decided to wait a few days before committing to the idea that I was depressed. I felt overwhelmed, exhausted and emotional, but I still felt giddy with love for my son, and didn't feel completely hopeless about my future, as uncertain as it still was.

And as the weeks passed, the emotional fog I was wandering about in did lift, and I began to feel a little more like myself.

About three weeks after Tor's birth, I woke up and felt different. It was a subtle change, but noticeable. As though I'd been semi-sedated the whole time, and the drugs had finally worn off, giving me back some energy and clarity. For the first time, I didn't lie in bed half-awake, wishing someone would beat me unconscious so I could have just a few more hours of rest. I slipped out of the sheets, stood up and walked over to the bassinet, where Tor was also waking from a four-hour sleep.

'Good morning, Buddy,' I said, gently picking his swaddled form up in my arms. His small body instantly relaxed as I held him to my shoulder.

The 13 kilos of baby weight I had gained was almost gone, having been eaten up my by nutritionally deprived post-partum body and converted into breast milk.

I'd adjusted to the bite-sized portions of sleep, and our family had settled into a more predictable routine. I'd started to get my appetite back, and the iced coffee habit had now been contained to a single, mini-sized bottle in the morning, followed by a more substantial breakfast of avocado and Vegemite on miche toast or a couple of hard-boiled eggs.

The change in my outlook was dramatic, and I felt much more confident about tackling the start of the new treatment.

But even though I felt more capable, and a little more lucid, I had no idea how mentally fragile I still really was.

◆ ◆ ◆

Tor had a wonky head. He had started favouring just one side when he slept, and by the time he was a few months old, he'd developed a flat spot on the left side of his soft skull. It wasn't dramatically obvious, but I could tell—and, while his dad still had a pretty good head of hair, as did my dad, if by chance the poor kid turned out follically challenged like his dad's dad I didn't want to be responsible for failing to correct his asymmetrical head.

So we took him to a specialist, to see if anything could be done before his skull hardened into its forever shape. The specialist, Brent, was a pleasantly spoken bloke in his early forties. We hit it off instantly, as he had an easy-going personality and was great with Tor. As we walked into his surgery a little girl, about the age of six, was leaving with her mum. She had cerebral palsy, and was walking with the aid of stirrups and crutches. 'I've identified a number of kids with it early on over the years,' he explained, as Tor and I sat down at his desk.

From his desk drawer, he took out a thick, white elastic band, which had red dots marked on it, and placed it on Tor's head, transforming him into a mini ninja. The band was a measuring tool to determine the extent of Tor's plagiocephaly—the medical term for wonky baby head syndrome. Tor's case was moderate. A few sessions would determine if Brent could stop it progressing and even it out more. Brent picked him up around his waist, then tilted his body to the right, and then to the left. 'Hmm, he's a little stronger on his left side,' he concluded.

'Is that normal?' I asked.

'Hmm, some kids develop on one side faster than the other,' he replied.

Tor's right neck and shoulder had stiffened since he'd started favouring the other side, so we were sent home with instructions to try to get him to look to the other side as much as possible.

Later that day I placed Tor on his change table to give him a fresh nappy. He had started lifting his left arm above his head, like he was giving the air a fist pump. He did it a couple of times as I changed him. *That's so cute,* I thought as I clipped his white onesie back on.

I then noticed that his right arm remained bent, his hand clenched into a tight fist. 'C'mon buddy, use the other hand,' I encouraged, lifting it up near his head. It shot back down like an elastic band. My heart started to beat faster, and a bolt of panic shot down my body as more thoughts of the little girl in Brent's surgery came to mind.

I didn't tell Nick my concerns about Tor's asymmetrical development that night when he came home, but I became hyper-alert to every single movement my baby made. He *did* favour his left side more than his right, I concluded. I told myself not to panic. *Just call Brent first thing tomorrow and ask him to tell you straight whether or not he thinks Tor has cerebral palsy.*

I hardly slept that night. My mind was plagued with thoughts of what our life might look like if he did have a disability. Of course I'd love him no matter what, but the notion crushed me with guilt. *What if my illness had something to do with it? What if it was the interferon injections?* I wondered as I lay in the dark. *Please God,* I silently begged as I stared up at the ceiling. *Throw whatever you want at me. Hurt me, maim me, kill me—but leave my baby alone.* I'd weathered the events of the past year with my sanity and hope still intact, but I knew I was just one more tragedy away from completely, and utterly, falling apart.

When I didn't hear back from Brent by 10 a.m. the next morning, I couldn't help but Google *early signs of cerebral palsy.*

Nick returned from his morning gym session to find me hysterically sobbing. I was sitting on the rug on the living room floor, clutching Tor in my arms and rocking him back and forth like a traumatised child with her doll.

'Elle, what's happened, are you ok? What's wrong with Tor?!' he said urgently. He threw his bag down on the step and rushed into the living room.

Tears were streaming down my face and I was hyperventilating. 'Tor's got cerebral palsy,' I managed to say. 'I'm sure of it.' I was stroking his head vigorously, as we sat on the floor of the living room, refusing to let go of his tiny, squirming body.

A look of realisation dawned on Nick's face. 'He does *not*, Elle!' Nick exclaimed. 'You've just worked yourself up into a frenzy—you need to calm down. You're being completely irrational. Have you called Brent?'

'He's not answering,' I replied. I handed Nick my phone, and told him to watch the YouTube video I'd found. The video showed a baby who, at about the same age as Tor, was favouring one side of his body, and had later been diagnosed with the condition. Nick finished watching the video, and stood up.

'For fuck's sake, Elle, you need to stop working yourself up like this. You've got no evidence and there's no point becoming hysterical from watching a bloody YouTube video.'

My phone rang a few minutes later, and fortunately by this stage Nick had managed to calm me down. It was Brent.

I relayed my fears to him as I paced our front lawn, and explained the reasons for my suspicions.

'Elle I'm so sorry if I gave you that impression,' he replied. 'I have absolutely no concern about Tor in that regard. A lot of babies' bodies develop this way; I'm sure in a few weeks his other side will catch up and there'll be no problem at all. There's honestly nothing to worry about.'

The relief made my legs weak. I sat down on the damp grass and put my left hand to my heart, which had been racing since the night before.

A few weeks later Tor started using his right arm, and my fears dropped away.

◆ ◆ ◆

In hindsight, my incessant worrying about Tor's health was a way to distract myself from the nervousness I felt about starting my treatment. Prof had chosen to put me on a drug called nilotinib. It had been approved for use in Australia in 2008, and was the second generation of tyrosine kinase inhibitors following the success of Gleevec, the first TKI to come on the market. I was to take two tablets, twice a day, and would need to fast for two hours before, and one hour after taking them.

Gleevec had been trialled in the late 1990s, when the outlook for people diagnosed with chronic myeloid leukaemia was grim. Before 2001, fewer than one in three patients with CML survived longer than five years after being first diagnosed. It was a death sentence, and the only chance to be cured involved a brutal, and risky, bone marrow transplant.

In 1998, a US doctor named Brian Druker began trialling Gleevec (generic name imatinib mesylate) on humans. The drug switched off the enzymes that caused the cancer, and was a resounding success. The outlook for patients once these drugs came on the market was overwhelmingly positive.

Had I started my treatment immediately after I had been diagnosed, there would have been almost no doubt in my mind that I would survive this disease. But waiting nine months untreated had changed the game for me. It would be a long time before I knew whether that delay in treatment would affect my ability to one day stop taking the drugs and remain in remission indefinitely.

Popping four pills daily sounded straightforward, but the more common side effects included fatigue, nausea, skin rashes, hair loss and bone pain. The drug could also affect the heart, liver and glucose balance, and cause a drop in blood counts. Among my Facebook forum buddies, skin issues were top of the list, alongside severe fatigue, 'chemo brain' and hair thinning.

A few days before I took my first dose of nilotinib, I bought six pink grapefruits and finished them all off. Grapefruit, one of my all-time favourite fruits, had been proven to interfere with absorption of the drug, so it would be off the menu indefinitely—but by the time I popped the first pair of little orange pills, I could barely look at a grapefruit after my citrus overdose.

'Cancer unicorn, I'm a cancer unicorn,' I kept repeating to myself, hoping for minimal side effects from my new treatment. After all, I'd coped with the interferon drugs just fine . . .

◆ ◆ ◆

You should STOP nilotinib completely for the moment. If you develop bleeding or a fever or other signs of infection, please contact me or the haematology unit at RPAH.

It wasn't the most heartening email to receive from Prof at 2 a.m. I'd been up feeding Tor when I heard the familiar *ping* of my email alert.

Just got your latest blood count result and it shows a further drop in both neutrophils and platelets, he wrote.

The late hour of the email and my drowsy head didn't help me absorb the email calmly and rationally.

My extremely low blood counts were concerning, as it predisposed me to infection and bleeding, Prof later explained. Since starting nilotinib a few weeks before, I'd developed a few side effects, but they were bearable. It was hard to know whether the fatigue was due to being a new mum or the drug, but I told myself it was definitely the former, because I was a cancer unicorn—one of the few who would sail through treatment and get back to living life.

But I couldn't ignore the changes to my skin. Within just a few days, my once smooth dermis had changed texture. I developed a rash on my calves and chest, and my face now felt as rough and bumpy as sandpaper. But how could I complain when other cancer sufferers could hardly walk from the fatigue of intravenous chemotherapy, and lost all their hair? I was so lucky that the drugs I had to take didn't require hours in the hospital. *It's a ridiculously small price to pay to stay alive, so be grateful for Christ's sake,* I'd tell myself most mornings as I washed my dry, gritty face.

A few months before giving birth, I visited my hairdresser, George Giavis, for a trim. I told him I'd be starting an oral chemotherapy drug the following year, and there was a chance I'd experience hair loss. 'It's not *all* going to fall out,' I assured him as he shampooed my hair in the porcelain basin. 'But my hair's not exactly thick now, so I'm preparing myself for the odd bald patch.'

'Trust me, honey, I've got some great contacts in the wig industry,' he promised, 'you'll look fabulous no matter what.'

I did lose a lot of hair in the months following treatment, but nothing a little teasing at the roots couldn't hide.

Prof advised me to stop taking the pills for a few weeks, until my blood counts reached more normal levels. I didn't like the idea of stopping treatment, as reaching remission was largely dependent on taking the drugs consistently—and a few missed doses could allow the cancer genes to mutate, making it resistant to treatment and reducing my chance of reaching total remission. But at least I could cram in a few more grapefruit binges.

One positive aspect was that the drug did seem to be effective against my cancer, with my BCR–ABL having dropped in the five weeks since I started taking it. The problem was, it was just working a little too well. When my blood counts normalised, Prof explained, we would try the drug again on a lower dosage. Eventually I'd increase my dosage to the same strength again, and hopefully my body would have learned to cope with it and I could remain on it without any further problems.

If not, then I'd still have a few more drug options left, thankfully. But as a cancer unicorn, I was hopeful Prof had chosen the right drug first off.

◆ ◆ ◆

In the days after I stopped taking nilotinib, my energy levels were noticeably higher. It was a relief not having to think about fasting, and not having to wake up at 5 a.m. to take my first dose of pills for the day.

A few weeks later, another blood test revealed my blood counts were returning to more normal levels. I started treatment again that same week, and aside from a fresh wave of exhaustion and a bad leg rash, I was feeling ok.

Video diary, 12 April 2017

Just went and saw the Prof and good news: my BCR–ABL level has dropped from 16 per cent down to 0.18 per cent, which is unbelievable. And all of my neutrophils—and white blood cells and platelets, and all of that—have all gone up, so they're pretty close to normal now, which is really good.

For a while it was looking a bit sketchy so I'm very, very happy and we're going to go out for breakfast at Bill's cafe today. I'm actually feeling a little under the weather, I'm getting a cold, I think.

But yeah, I'm still celebrating. I'm pretty happy and all is well. Bye!

Happy Cancerversary

Is it a day of mourning? A day to reflect on the life you once had before your identity was ripped away and replaced by another? Or do you celebrate? Pop a bottle of champagne, blow up a few balloons and pat yourself on the back for staying alive for another year?

On my cancerversary I felt torn between the two.

The day prior I'd attended my cousin's wedding. My sisters Amy and Martine and their families had flown down from

Queensland to attend the nuptials, which were held at the Hydro Majestic, in the Blue Mountains. My dad was there, with Suzette, and all of my aunties, uncles and cousins.

The weather was absolutely perfect, and the day went without a hitch. It felt so good to be surrounded by my family that day—to be celebrating love, and the promise of a happy future for a young couple.

I woke up the next day at sunrise with a huge smile on my face. For all the pain and worry the past year had brought, I had many more things to be happy and grateful for.

I crept over to the small bassinet at the base of our bed, where our five-month-old son was still quietly sleeping. He had started sleeping through the night at three months and, after an unsettled period at the four-month mark, had returned to pulling those blessed all-nighters.

I wish I could say I had become completely and utterly enlightened during my cancer and pregnancy journey. That I never lost my temper, that small inconveniences or 'First World problems' no longer irritated me, and that my day-to-day life was a perfectly balanced, Instagram-worthy pyramid of meditation, green smoothies and mindfulness.

I still stress out if I'm running late for an appointment, or I burn dinner. I still get impatient with my husband over unnecessary things, and I still down the occasional glass (or two) of red wine after particularly trying days of baby-wrangling. But the feelings pass more quickly now. I forgive myself faster, laugh things off and refuse to spend time mulling over what I now call 'micro-dramas'.

According to the Cancer Council, 68 per cent of Australians are still alive five years after a cancer diagnosis.

For a number of those survivors, cancer profoundly alters their futures. Some stop smoking, others become more sun smart, and some use the diagnosis as a wake-up call to work less, spend more time with loved ones, tick off things on their bucket lists and finally have the courage to pursue their dreams.

For others, it's a reason to wallow in self-pity. Some drink more, abuse prescription painkillers, make risky life choices. Some even live life exactly as they had before their diagnosis.

I'm not one of that 68 per cent who is still alive five years after a cancer diagnosis. Not yet. But I'm hopeful, and confident, as are my doctors, that I will reach that milestone.

It's even possible that I could celebrate my five-year cancer-versary by trying for another baby. But that's a long way away, and something I'm not yet ready to consider.

I live more simply now. I've stopped accumulating things in the hope it will bring me closer to a perfect, happy life. I give more thought to my purchases, and try to buy only things I need, rather than want.

I've finally realised it's futile to chase happiness in the form of things and objects. As children, it was so easy to believe that once you had that toy/game/scooter you had been pestering your parents about for weeks, life would be complete. *The moment I get it in my hot little hand,* you would repeatedly tell yourself, *I will never want for anything again.*

For many of us, the objects of desire change as we get older, but the same mentality remains. It's inevitable, however, that before long that bigger house will become too small, the new car will lose its shine and the designer handbag will become worn and outdated.

In the months following my pregnancy I did a lot of soul searching. Slowly I began to consider my diagnosis not as a tragedy, but a second shot at living the best, most authentic life that I could. A life that would make me proud.

Did I want to be remembered for my shoe collection or my attendance at red carpet parties? I asked myself more than once. No. *Did anyone I cared about give a damn whether I had a large social media following?* I hoped not.

A few weeks before my cancerversary I sat down with a pen and paper, and for the first time, wrote down a list of my values.

It was quickly apparent, as I jotted them down, that up until April 2016 my life had been completely misaligned with these values. No wonder I had battled anxiety for so many years. I'd been swimming against a current of perfection and was simply exhausted.

Animal welfare was high on the list of causes I held dear. But I owned two fur coats, because they were fashionable. I valued spending time with my loved ones, yet over the years I had missed weddings, birthday parties and even funerals in favour of work. I valued spending time in nature, yet most of my days had been spent in an office or a shopping centre. Honesty was another big one, but how many times had I ignored my own feelings in order to be the nice, polite girl who fitted in with the crowd?

It was incredibly hard to be so brutally transparent with myself. Guilt, regret and fear were just a couple of the emotions I felt as I looked back at my twenties and the energy I'd wasted trying to be someone else. Someone who, when I really thought about it, I didn't like.

I put down my pen, walked into my bedroom and opened my wardrobe cupboard. I pulled out the black fur gilet I'd been given for my 27th birthday, and a vintage leather jacket with a fox fur collar. The next morning I drove into the car park at Woolworth's supermarket in Balmain, and put the furs into one of the red Salvos store's charity bins.

Cancer has taught me that life is not to be lived perfectly. We all fuck up. We all do dumb things, hurt people we love, and say the wrong things out of anger, or frustration, or fear. We waste time, waste money, and consume more than we need. We care too much about what other people think, we avoid doing things that scare us, and we forget how important it is to stop sometimes and be grateful for our lot in life.

But I've learned that imperfection is okay, as long as everything we do comes from a place of love. Love is what got me through my diagnosis, and what helped me to make a choice no woman should have to make in her lifetime.

A mother's love is more powerful than I could have ever imagined.

30 April 2017

Dear Tor,
One year ago today you made yourself known. You were barely more than a few cleverly assembled cells but were growing by the minute. You scared me. I wasn't sure if we would both make it, but we did.

You're nearly five months old now. You have the rosiest cheeks, and I reckon you're just a few weeks away from getting your very first tooth.

It's been a learning curve for your dad and me. I've only just started to feel confident that I can tell your hungry cry from your tired cry. Thanks for being patient.

I wonder if you're going to be interested in reading these emails when you're old enough to do so. Perhaps this email address will be forgotten, and join the other million defunct addresses (like my very first one which was something like sochic007@hotmail.com—I know, at the dawn of the internet we didn't have a clue!) floating around the net.

But on the off chance you are interested in knowing about your first year on Earth, here are some of your quirks which make us laugh and love you more and more each day:

Your favourite song is 'Agadoo', the 80s hit by Black Lace (stops you crying every time).

You look like Astro Boy right now, thanks to your very pronounced widow's peak. Nobody can figure out who you inherited that from!

A navy-blue bunny rabbit and a monkey blanket made by Doctor Don's partner Mora are your favourite toys, but they are now having to compete with Chairman Meow for attention, as his fluffy tale is proving irresistible to your curious hands.

You've just started to taste real food, and so far you're pretty much into every type of vegetable we give you. Unfortunately you've also learned to blow raspberries, which you love to practise with said solids in your mouth. It makes for good videos though.

You love people, and look to be following in your dad's footsteps when it comes to socialising. But I'm clearly your favourite; your beaming smile when I pick you up each morning tells me so.

I can't wait to see you take your first steps, say your first words, make your first friend at kindergarten and pursue your dreams when you grow up. But I can wait, because I love you as you are, right here, right now, blowing raspberries on my shoulder and grasping my arm with your tiny, perfect hand.

With love forever, and ever, no matter what happens.

Your mum,
Elle

Hope Shines Bright

6 October 2017

I felt nervous as I ascended the steps onto the temporary stage at Sydney's Barangaroo Reserve and gripped the microphone. The Leukaemia Foundation had invited me to become an ambassador and emcee for their 2017 Light the Night fundraising walk, a year after I had first taken part in the event, and I had instantly said 'yes'.

Having hosted countless events in front of huge groups of people, I was surprised to have so many butterflies in my gut as I welcomed the crowd of thousands to the annual walk with J.Mo, who had agreed to co-host. But tonight was different. I wasn't introducing celebrities or discussing the latest beauty range. I was speaking to hundreds of people who, in many ways, were my heroes. Through their donations and support, they were helping Australians and their families who were dealing with a blood cancer diagnosis.

I scanned the crowd and found Nick, who was holding Tor. The pair were surrounded by dozens of our friends and family, who were all holding blue lanterns to signal their support.

Nick smiled and gave me a subtle nod of encouragement. I took a deep breath in, and relaxed my shoulders.

'Many of you are here to remember loved ones lost, and there are others here who stand alongside someone you know affected by blood cancer,' I began. 'By walking together and raising funds, we light the way for those 35 Australians diagnosed today, showing them they're not alone.'

I asked the sea of people to light their blue, gold or white lanterns and raise them high. Suddenly the park was illuminated by hundreds of soft coloured lights.

'Your gold lantern represents a special person who is no longer here, but you hold in your heart,' I continued.

'Your white lantern is a symbol of your own personal blood cancer experience. It reflects the hope of making a better future for those who may have to follow in your footsteps.'

'Blue is the colour of the Leukaemia Foundation and represents how, together, we can be the light in the darkest hour for people in our community devastated by a blood cancer diagnosis.'

I asked the crowd to turn around to face the banner at the start of the walk, which weaved around the foreshore of Sydney Harbour. 'Now, let's walk together to Light the Night.'

Nick was waiting for me as the crowd began to make its way along the waterfront. Tor was moments away from sleep in his pram, and I had to fight the urge to pick him up and hug him. I gave Nick a kiss.

'You did great, Ellie,' he assured me. 'I'm really proud of you.'

17 October 2017

Mathematics was never my strong point at high school. I dropped maths classes in Year 10, and freely admit I've never found myself in a situation that required me to remember even the basic algebra I learned. But I know enough to realise that the percentage I'm staring at in Doc's office is significant: 0.0071 per cent.

It's the result of my latest blood test, and the number is the percentage of cancerous BCR–ABL genes currently detectable in my blood.

I'm in deep molecular remission. I'm winning the battle.

My BCR–ABL had steadily decreased in the months following the start of my treatment, but this latest result is a milestone.

My heart skips a beat and I give Tor, who is perched on my lap studying his toy caterpillar, an excited squeeze. Nick is sitting next to us, with a huge grin on his face. He still comes to every appointment, and I love him for it.

If my remission stays on course for the next three to four years, I'll be well placed to consider stopping my drug therapy indefinitely.

It would mean the end of three-hour fasting sessions and drug-induced daily fatigue. *Life would go back to normal*, I think as we walk back to our car after the appointment.

Except that it won't. My future had irrevocably changed 18 months ago, and I can never go back to being the person I was before. And I don't want to, either.

I have less energy now, and I'm sure there will be moments when I wish I could erase the c-word from my medical records. Will I be considered a liability to potential employers? Will I age faster and be susceptible to other health problems as I get older? It's too early to know.

But for now, those questions can wait. In contrast to the events of the previous year, my life has regained some semblance of normality. I'm back at *The Daily Telegraph*, covering fashion, and like many women my age, trying to balance my career with motherhood.

I've recommenced my nutrition studies with renewed enthusiasm, this time with the goal of pairing this knowledge with what I've learned through my personal challenges in the hope of inspiring people to lead a healthier and more authentic life.

I'm more attuned to my body, and as a result have developed a beautiful relationship with it. I look after it, with regular yoga classes, rest, meditation and a wholefoods and probiotic-based diet.

I also take care of my mind, which is now free of the debilitating anxiety it was once plagued with. I still worry, of course, but it's usually fleeting, and without the sweaty palms, breathlessness and self-doubt. The nasty inner voice that constantly told me I was never good enough has been replaced by a new one—a voice that is much more forgiving, loving and kind.

A Mother's Choice

As I place Tor in his car seat, my inner voice pipes up. It reminds me I still have to drop my prescription to the pharmacy. *You also have to send that parcel to your sister before 6 p.m. and take the washing off the line . . .*

I blow Tor a raspberry. He giggles, and blows me one back.

Don't bother me now, I tell that inner voice. *I'm in the middle of something much more important.*

Acknowledgements

To Nick, thank you for holding my hand through the challenges and triumphs of these past two years and for continuing to do so as our hands become arthritic, age-spotted and wrinkled.

Het and Pete, who without your combined support, love and babysitting services, this book would not exist.

To my mum, for your sacrifices, for giving me faith in the universe that it will all work out, and for your unwavering love and dedication to your daughters and our children.

To my dad. Cancer can be a lonely illness, but having someone to whinge to and swap war stories with, and who understands what you're going through, has been a huge comfort. I love you so much.

To Suzette, for your magic baby-whispering skills, keeping me so well fed during marathon writing sessions and offering no-nonsense life advice.

Thank you, Doctor Donny. Your thorough medical care and smart-arse jokes kept me alive and laughing through the whole ordeal. Seriously, we're so grateful to have you in our lives.

To Prof. Your knowledge and expertise have been invaluable; thanks for being patient with us, answering all of our sometimes inane questions and guiding us through some of the tough moments of my cancer treatment and pregnancy.

Thanks to Tim Hughes and the team at SAHMRI. You've been incredibly supportive. Thanks for working so hard to find a cure.

To Claire, Tom, Siobhán, Patrizia and the awesome team at Allen & Unwin, for allowing me to share my story, and believing that I could raise two babies simultaneously even if I didn't believe it myself. And (in advance!) for your patience. Your incredible patience.

Lauren, for taking a chance on me and giving me the confidence to write this book; your sage advice and motivational chats helped me more than you know.

To Bianca, for capturing Tor and me so beautifully in the cover shot.

To my beautiful sisters Amy, Martine and Chrissy: I don't need to explain how much I love you. And Angus, my brother from another mother!

To the friends who called or texted just to check in, when I needed it the most. You know you who are.

To Granny, for raising such a wonderful family and showing so much strength and resilience. You are an amazing woman.

To my cousins, aunties and uncles: I'm so proud to call myself a Halliwell; I couldn't have wished for a more awesome bunch of relos. A special thanks to the Stevens family; Natalie's strength was my guiding light and you are doing an amazing job continuing her legacy.

To my seniors at News Corp. I'm eternally grateful for your support and flexibility as I acclimatised to my new situation.

Thanks to Stef, Ally and the *60 Minutes* team for sharing my story and raising awareness for CML. Ally, I'm so blessed to now call you a friend.

And to my son, Tor Felix. You are my miracle, my world and my reason for everything.